YOU HAVE SUCH A PRETTY FACE

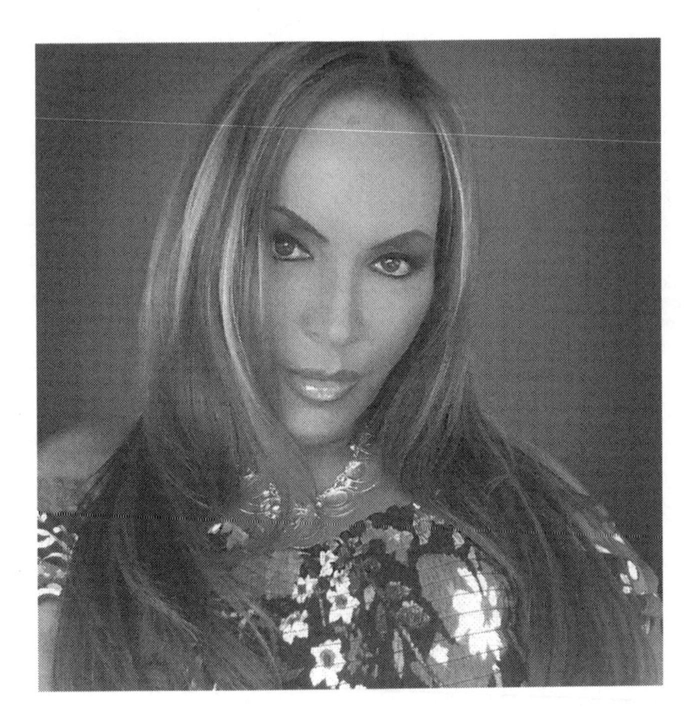

YOU HAVE SUCH A PRETTY FACE

A Memoir of Trauma, Hope,
and the Joy that Follows Survival

KELLEY GUNTER

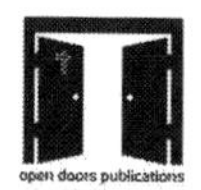

Published by Open Doors Publishing, 2017

Cover and interior design by Damonza

Cover Photo by Lori Hughes

Preliminary edits, Sarah Butler
Full edit, Holly Jordan

ISBN-13: 978-0692936818 (Custom Universal)
ISBN-10: 0692936815

Printed and bound in the United States of America

This book is written for my son, Alec, and my best friend, Lori, who both, at one time or another, have:

1. Held my hair when I vomited
2. Grabbed ice cream when I cried
3. Laughed with me and AT me until we peed, (okay, until I peed)
4. Accompanied me on my search for the world's best homemade desserts
5. Believed in me when I'd lost belief in myself
6. Celebrated me at my best
7. Loved me at my worst
8. Prayed with me
9. Stood firm when the rest of the world walked out
10. Been my biggest blessing

To say I love you simply doesn't cover it.
My cup runneth over.
XOXO

PROLOGUE

I DON'T KNOW everything.

I don't even know a lot.

But I do know some things, and this is what I know for sure:

You are not reading this by accident.

This book has made its way into your hands for a reason. It's funny how life works like that. I don't believe in chance or coincidences—I have always believed that coincidences are small miracles where God has chosen to remain anonymous. God has intervened anonymously in my life so many times, and when I have allowed myself to receive the message that was being presented to me, it usually resulted in some pretty incredible outcomes. That's not to say that the path was always easy, but that the final destination was worth the journey. So, whether you believe in God or the Universe or a Higher Power, whatever your beliefs, this book has ended up with you for a reason.

Either you or someone you care about is struggling with a weight issue. It's a journey I have embarked upon and a pain I have known well. It's a pain unlike any other, an inescapable feeling of a multitude of emotions, all of them hurtful and filled with despair. I spent many years walking down that path and when I speak to or see others who are currently navigating that incredibly difficult terrain, I stop, pause, and remember, "I've been there."

This book is meant to tell a bigger story than just weight loss. It's a story about survival, struggle, love, heartbreak, determination, happiness, and faith. Once I had achieved my weight loss, I took off running toward life with open arms. I was eager to embrace the world without the restraints of an extra 243 pounds. Still, God kept reminding me to tell this story. He kept tapping me on the shoulder as if to say, "I kept you here for a reason. Your survival was intentional."

So now, I'm telling that story.

"When the world says, 'give up,'
Hope whispers, 'try it one more time.'"

—Unknown

PART I

"What I am looking for is not out there, it is in me."

—Helen Keller

CHAPTER 1

H.O.P.E.

Hold On, Pain Ends.

We live in a world full of survivors. The walking wounded are everywhere and I was one of them. I have the heart of a survivor, one that has been walked on, broken, used, and disregarded many times. I'm guessing—in fact I'm pretty certain—that you, too, have such a heart. It is impossible to have walked this particular path and not have endured the hurts that earn you the right to wear that badge.

I have a plethora of experiences, stories and scars. I've been knee deep in emotional battle and lived through psychological combat intense enough that when it was all said and done, I wondered if it would have been smarter to have surrendered. But as I emerged from the ruins of what I once thought was my safe haven, I couldn't help but have the unmistakable presence and shine of a warrior after battle; the last one standing, if you will; the swagger of a winner who knows—I made it through the rain. It's a title I wear with a sense of shame or pride, depending on the day. Surviving is the quintessential double-edged sword—a weapon that at one point or another, I would have been happy to use to cut the tongue out of the callous and heartless person who just asked me if I weighed a ton.

Because I've been there, I can say that sometimes life is very difficult and can be filled with pain. I've learned that life doesn't always play fair or play by any set of rules at all. As babies, we certainly didn't get to choose the bodies we were born into and the genetics we were assigned. I've heard it said that our physical bodies are just the "house" for our souls while we are on this earth. If that's the case, then I would've liked to have been born with a nice, little, middle-of-the-road, average house for my soul to inhabit while here. I didn't need a mansion or anything fancy: normalcy was enough. Just average would have been fine. I feel that I was placed into a house that ultimately fell apart, turned on me like a poltergeist had taken it over, and finally was found to be deplorable and was condemned.

My journey was not a quick one. I had an average body as I grew up. Throughout high school I played sports and was active, but I was also always trying to lose weight to be as small as my friends. I can't remember a time in high school that I was happy with my body or that I wasn't dieting to try to get into better shape. It was a constant struggle. I honestly can't even remember a time when I wasn't on some sort of diet. This pattern continued throughout college as well, where I began gaining more weight. Once I had graduated, the weight piled on in a fairly quick fashion. In short, I was always the big girl. In spite of never liking my body to begin with, once I had gained a significant amount of weight, I would look back at old pictures and think that I wasn't really that big back then and I'd wish I could be that size again.

Haven't we all done that? We look at old pictures and wish we could be back there? We might even keep those old pictures up, have them on our desk at work or out at home. We might use an old picture as our Facebook profile picture, one that shows us thinner and happier. By doing so, we are, in effect, "proving" ourselves. People can see who we once were, and we hope it softens how they see us in the present.

I did this all the time. I proudly displayed who I used to be, never letting on that when I was that person, I wasn't happy in that body. I find that fact interesting and enlightening now, but we will jump off of that bridge in a few chapters. People would ask who that was in my old pictures and when I would say that it was me, they were astonished. I guess those pictures were my way of letting everyone know that I wasn't always this big. In my mind, I thought if they knew that I used to be smaller they might like me better or accept me more easily. I thought men I might be interested in dating would find me more desirable if they knew I used to be thinner. Maybe they would be interested in me if they thought there was hope in me being smaller again. I built my confidence on a past daydream that had never existed in the first place, but it was all that I could do. Because even when I was the girl in the pictures, I wasn't happy with my body.

It's fascinating how our mind bargains with the truth like that. It's an escape mechanism that assists us in dealing with our painful reality for the time being. As a licensed social worker, I already knew that escapism is never healthy, but that never stopped me from using it myself. Negotiating with life about who we are based on how we look, is like being the Homecoming Queen of Crazy Town. No one wants to be that girl. I mean yes, there *is* a tiara involved, but no one really wants to wear that crown.

In reality, I didn't think I was okay being a bigger person. The truth behind that escapism was this: I would sit at the mirror and look at myself, thinking, "Why are you even bothering to do your makeup? You're just a four-hundred-pound woman and people will see right through you, makeup won't make you beautiful when the whole world thinks you're ugly." Now, equipped with 20/20 hindsight, I see that my soul wasn't happy and I desperately needed some version of hope to grasp onto until I figured out a way to slay the monster inside that controlled me.

Those old pictures didn't serve as motivation for me, however. Instead, they were a quiet reminder of who I once was. I would silently wish I could somehow go back in time to be that girl again, even knowing that I wasn't happy with that body either. That mindset didn't make any sense, but I utilized it regularly. See, we are back to that Homecoming Queen I spoke of earlier. Yes, I was reigning over Crazy Town, in spite of the fact that I was missing my tiara.

The truth is, I wanted to be in shape. I wanted to turn heads when I walked into a room, and I wanted to find a man who really thought I was beautiful. Most importantly, I wanted to think I was beautiful. I wanted to be healthy. I was missing my life. I would decline invitations because I knew I couldn't physically handle the activity. And if I could, I didn't want to embarrass myself by being the fat girl who looked funny or couldn't perform well.

After college, I could hardly imagine being capable of going to the clubs or bars with my friends, and when I did, I imagined myself sitting at the bar alone while all the other girls got hit on, checking over my shoulder for people laughing if I decided to dance, and spending the night trying to ignore the rude comments. All of these things had happened to me in the past, and they didn't feel good. Trust me when I tell you that it is not fun to be the young, heavy girl who sits alone all night and watches all of the attractive, young men approach her friends.

People had laughed at me for years. It's intensely strange how people laugh at those who are hurting. I didn't bother people. When I was out, I stuck with my friends and I didn't try to draw attention to myself. Nonetheless, there was always someone who would have to make some snide comment at my expense. Everyone around would hear it and laugh and miss the sadness in my eyes when I heard the comment, too. They would miss the tears that streamed down my face as I walked away. How was I supposed to respond? There wasn't anything I could have said.

Once, when a man had started to flirt with me at a sporting event, his friend said that he was called the "Milkman" because he only dated cows. I remember everyone laughing. I was trying to hold the tears back, but eventually they began to spill over. As I turned to leave, I heard the man comment that maybe I should go eat another gallon of ice cream and cry by myself.

Who actually says those kinds of things to a complete stranger or to anyone at all? When I was growing up, my Grandmother, who we called Nonnie, (remember that name, you'll hear it again), always told me that saying someone else is ugly doesn't make you any prettier. Apparently, many of the people I've encountered in my life missed that memo. I really don't believe that people want to be hurtful. I choose to believe that most people, one on one, would not be that way. But group mentality can be vicious. The sad truth is that being a big person makes you an easy target for mean, callous, ignorant people who have no problem vying for attention by getting others to laugh at someone else's expense. I absorbed those words like a bacteria until they turned suffering into sickness. All of those words, hurts, all of those tears, were forever etched into my heart. When I remember that pain, I think back to my childhood when I was taught that "sticks and stones will break my bones but words will never harm me." I tend to agree more with the words of Robert Fulghum:

"Sticks and stones will break my bones, but words will break my heart."

CHAPTER 2

"Be careful what you say.
You can say something hurtful in ten seconds,
But ten years later,
The wounds are still there.

—Joel Osteen

The human spirit can be fragile and easily endure irreparable damage. Hurtful words can penetrate your soul and find a permanent resting place in the shallows of an already aching heart. While there were so many facets to the pain of being overweight, one of the most painful for me was the words spoken to me and about me.

It always surprises me that in spite of how far I've come, I haven't been able to permanently delete the painful words from my memory. It would be nice if my heart had an "empty trash bin" button like my computer, so I could just erase those hurtful things forever. But the mind, the heart, and the soul don't operate in that fashion.

It is important to understand, however, that perhaps the pain of those hurtful words needs to be remembered for a reason. Even today as I remember the hurtful things that were said to me, I can still feel some of the pain and sadness. I'm instantly transported back to those moments and I've never forgotten how it felt. Honestly, I don't ever want to forget how it felt. There's a reason that I'm able to feel so deeply the pain that others feel, and there is a reason that I have deep empathy for others—I have experienced heartbreak, too.

When I was in junior high and high school, I was a cheerleader. During one game, I saw some of the boys in the stands looking at me and laughing. Later on the bus ride home, someone called me "Richter." I didn't know what that meant. I eventually found out that the cruel nickname referred to the Richter Scale—the scale that expresses the magnitude of an earthquake. Of course, the name stuck and boys would call me that as I walked down the school hallway, and everyone would laugh at my expense. I remember going home, telling my mom, and crying all night long. I felt betrayed by the mockery coming from these people who were supposedly my friends, even close friends at that.

Another name they stuck me with was "Tree Trunk Legs." Self-explanatory, uncreative, but even still, devastating. I can remember two of my so-called friends writing notes back and forth during science class. Somehow the note ended up in my hands. I remember it so clearly that I can feel myself back in the same classroom. My "friends" had been drawing cartoon pictures of me with tree trunks for legs. Again, that was another name that stayed with me for years, drawing laughter from everyone. If I answered a question incorrectly in class, one of the guys would say something like, "Shut up Tree Trunks," or "Don't you know the answer, Richter?" It was torture if one of my friends would be angry with me, because they would know just the right names to use to hurt me intentionally.

We all know it well: high school teenagers are cruel. I went to a small school in southern Ohio with the typical cliques of girls and guys. They would all turn on someone when they were upset, and I was an easy target. It didn't help that my very best friend and I didn't have a single class together. It would probably surprise my former classmates to know how hurtful those comments were to me and how they are still clear in my mind today. Many people back then probably thought that I took it all in stride and laughed it off. Those people had to be blind or stupid. Perhaps both.

Clearly, my former classmates were blind and oblivious, and perhaps apathetic, to my pain and hurt. To be honest, I think they knew their words would hurt, but they just didn't care. I can remember a time when I sat at my desk with my head down, crying and thinking, "I cannot make it 'til graduation." I was filled with sadness and despair.

If you're reading this, if something similar has brought you to your knees, then you'll understand what I mean when I say that pain recognizes pain. I know your pain. I may not ever be able to remove someone else's pain, but Nonnie always told me, "A burden shared is a burden divided." When people share their pain with me, I hope and believe they can look into my eyes and see instantly that I am a fellow survivor. I hope they connect beyond my eyes and in that moment, say, "Ahhhhh, she's in the club."

Immediately, their soul is at ease. Isn't that a beautiful moment? We've all had ones like it at some point. That divine intervention, if you will, when we encounter a comrade to our soul. We find them in the most unrecognizable places and people. It's as if there's a secret handshake of the heart, a silent message in the eyes, an invisible connection of two souls. A soul unmistakably recognizes compassion and in that true acceptance, it finds a bridge to peace. I've journeyed across that bridge and hope to lead many others to that beautiful path as well. I believe that's why I am here. Most of my life would not make sense if that isn't true.

I was crying to my friend Darci one day and told her about the hurtful situation I was facing at school. We all have those rare, special people who appear in our lives and who help guide us through incredibly life-altering moments. My person, at that point in my life, was my friend Darci. We had been friends since kindergarten and because of her, I was able to separate myself from that unhealthy group of kids.

In our conversation, Darci talked me into changing my class schedule to the college prep tract, which would remove me from the "friends" who tormented me so. The day is still vivid to me: Darci stood by me and told me that I didn't need to be around people who treated me poorly, and that they were not real friends. She even walked upstairs to the guidance office with me, and we changed my schedule right then. It was a little scary because even though those friends mistreated me, they were familiar to me, and when they were being nice to me I had fun with them. I'd learned to accept their behavior because it was a comfortable, known entity. I was worried about losing them, and I was worried that they would be angry with me. When they were angry, life wasn't easy.

Do you recognize what persona I was taking on with my irrational thinking? Let me grab my crown because I'm back on my throne, reigning over Crazy Town again. People who care about you should never intentionally hurt you. Friends shouldn't make you cry by calling you names and making fun of your body. When we're insecure about who we are and when we don't feel worthy of anything better, we tolerate abuse because we have limited choices. Deep inside we don't feel like we are worthy of more. We're hurting, and therefore we take what we think is our only option. Sadly, for me, this particular high school experience repeated itself throughout adulthood. Some lessons need to be taught more than once before they are learned.

However, things can change. Thanks to Darci, my life took a dramatic turn for the better. A voice of reason, she even prepared me and told me that those same "friends" would start calling me to ask why I wasn't around anymore. Darci told me to not take their calls, or return them. And that's exactly what I did.

The rest of my high school years were far happier. I've never forgotten that day and I have never forgotten that girl. Darci was a life-changer and I still love her to this day, even though I haven't seen her in years. At a crucial, dark journey of my soul, an angel appeared, providing guidance, support, and light. The Bible states in Hebrews 13:2, "Be not forgetful to entertain strangers: for thereby some have entertained angels unawares." Angels come in all shapes and sizes and show up when you least expect them. At that point in my life, mine stood 5'4" tall and was a beautiful, blue-eyed blonde named Darci. She had a heart of gold then and stepped up and fought a battle for me without even knowing it. I am beyond thankful for her presence in my life at that time.

Even though I will always see Darci as an angel during those times, that's not to vilify those other people who were cruel to me. I would hope that they all grew into wonderful adults, and I would guess that they don't even realize how much their words hurt. But wouldn't it be wonderful if they did? Wouldn't it be fabulous if they raised children who didn't bully other kids in that manner? I know that I raised my son to be the defender of other children who couldn't defend themselves. I raised him to know that often in similar situations, if just one person speaks up and says, "Hey, that's not cool..." the tormenter will stop.

For me, my experiences came full circle in a positive way when, not that long ago, I ran into a young lady who had graduated high school with my son. She asked me if he still wanted to be President of the United States one day. Before I could even answer, she said that he should be, because he always spoke up for the kids who couldn't or didn't speak up for themselves. She said he always looked out for everybody. Nothing ever made me feel so proud in all of my life.

I went home and told my son about the conversation, and he just smiled. He had been in school with this girl since kindergarten and she had encountered a lot of adversity at a young age. As a result, she had not had an easy life. I was proud to know that my son had done what I had always instructed him to do and surprisingly he had never even told me of any of those situations. Because of my own hurt, I had raised a child who had possibly prevented or lessened someone else's pain, at least a couple of times. Hot damn and hallelujah! The Queen did something right!!! Where's my crown ?!

Even though the rest of my high school days were far more peaceful, cruelty is formed from a lack of empathy, which is founded in ignorance. Ignorance is capable of thriving in all stages of life, as I learned when I entered the workforce. A former boss of mine was sitting in a staff meeting with all of us, telling us that a woman she had just seen at a meeting had gained a significant amount of weight. She went on and on about how HUGE the woman was and then she looked at me, in front of the entire staff, and she said, "I swear to God she's as big as Kelley." I could have died. I was sitting there minding my own business and out of nowhere, I was hit with a comment that felt like a slap in the face.

Later, a co-worker of mine went to our boss and told her that her comment had really hurt my feelings and embarrassed me. My boss's response was that I was too sensitive. The next day when she came into the office and I was walking up the hall she commented, "Oh there's Kelley, Miss Sensitive Butt." Instead of apologizing to me or trying to understand how her words had hurt me, she instead chose to blame her hurtful comments on my sensitivity.

Another time at the same place of employment, my coworkers were discussing what they were wearing to a formal event. One of them asked me what my dress looked like, and before I could answer, another coworker said, "Oh, nobody cares what big ol' dress Kelley is wearing." Again, I was minding my own business when the verbal onslaught came my way. Incidents such as these leave a burning memory that is impossible to forget.

I share these stories because I think they illustrate perfectly how other people are simply ignorant and blind to the pain they cause through their flippant comments and actions. If someone has never been in the boxing ring, they don't know how much a punch hurts. But those random comments do hurt. They're a blow to an already staggering opponent.

A heavy friend of mine said to me one time that thin people will just never understand how it feels to be overweight, and as a result they say things that are very hurtful. Many people who have never struggled with a weight issue have no idea how much their words hurt. Those words can pummel the heart of someone fighting desperately to fit into a world where thin is not only expected, but idolized. However, people who fail to understand how it feels to be heavy don't corner the market on hurtful comments. Plenty of heavy people are also guilty of saying hurtful comments to or about other heavy people. As we've all heard before, "hurt people, hurt people." My hope would be that ALL people could begin to understand that words are powerful and can be very healing or hurtful.

The damage people cause with their words is harsh and surprising. But sometimes, well-meaning people end up hurting us, too, through their own attempts at being helpful. These are the people who ask when our baby is due, or how long ago we gave birth, or any other number of outrageous questions or comments. No one ever stops to consider that maybe we're not pregnant and have not recently given birth at all. These people don't stop to think that assuming so is crossing a boundary they do not have permission to walk over.

My personal favorite accidental insult—though that's quite the oxymoron—is the tried and true, "You have such a pretty face." I must have heard that one a thousand times if I heard it once. It came in different forms. Once, a good friend was talking to me about dieting and she mentioned that her mother said that it was just such a shame because, "Kelley has such a pretty face." I'm not sure of her intent behind this, but I'm here to let you know it didn't help me at all. What's the shame? Was my life a total loss because I wasn't packaged in a way she found attractive? Was my existence pointless? Why does weight alone make my life, "such a shame?"

Even when friends would try to set me up on a blind date, they would describe me as having "a very pretty face." Since everyone says it, let's explore the comment. What is the latent sentiment behind it? Obviously, this phrase indicates that the body is a mess. The body is not pretty. In fact, the body is ugly. Perfect strangers would meet me and tell me that I had such a pretty face. Even the lady at the checkout line would say it. Of course, it never feels like a compliment. Maybe I'm a "sensitive butt" as my past boss called me, but when I hear that phrase, I always hear that silent disclaimer screaming loudly, "You are fat! Your body is ugly! It's such a shame, but hey, you have a pretty face!" When I would express this to my friends they would tell me that I should learn to take it as a compliment.

But anyone who has heard this statement knows the hurtfulness behind it.

Because this is one of my tender spots, I must continue to explore this a little further. Let's think about any attractive female celebrity. Does anyone ever say, "She has such a pretty face?" No, they say she's beautiful. Plain and simple. She's gorgeous. She's lovely. She's pretty. No one ever says, "She has such a pretty face." Likewise, no one ever says, "he has such a handsome face." They say that he's handsome. This is all because in the eyes of most of the world, fat is not pretty, beautiful, handsome, or gorgeous. It really stinks, but that's just the truth. That's the world we live in.

If I told every story for each time I had been told, "You have such a pretty face," I would have to write an entire encyclopedia. One time someone said this to me during a telephone conversation and I was so annoyed, disgusted, and fed up with hearing the phrase that I walked out into my front yard and screamed at the heavens. No words, just a scream from the depths of my soul while shaking my fists wildly at the sky. Thank God my neighbors were my parents. They already knew about my throne and my crownless reign. I looked next door and my mom and dad happened to be sitting on their front porch. I looked down at the ground, shook my head, and thought to myself, "Oh great, let me go hear what this woman has to say." My mom, just like my Nonnie, always had the best one liners in the world. I walked over into their yard, sat down on the porch and my mom, who was my wise old owl said, "Let me guess, someone said you have such a pretty face?"

Because of my experiences, I make sure never to attach a qualifier to my compliment of an overweight person. Instead, I say, "You are so beautiful," or, "You are so handsome." Their eyes always light up, and it makes their day. Accordingly, it is important to make it a point never to tell people that a color or a dress looks nice on them. Make your compliments personal. Say, "You look so pretty in yellow," or, "You look so pretty in that dress." Don't say, "That's a beautiful dress." See the difference? Start incorporating that difference in your compliments. You'll see a difference in people's reactions. With that one little, simple adjustment, you have the power to make someone's day.

So, this is a challenge issued to all the people in the world reading this book. Please start telling bigger people that they are pretty, beautiful, handsome, PERIOD. Start realizing how you use your words. Start using your words with kindness and make a difference in someone's life in a positive way. Take it from me, I remember the kind and beautiful words spoken to me as much as I remember the hurtful ones. Words can be like magic. Think of the last time someone gave you a wonderful compliment or said something very nice. Didn't you replay it in your mind later? Maybe a thousand times?

Please walk gently through the life of another. I'm sure

you will find many worn out paths, some of which may look familiar and even hold your own footprints. As you walk along dreams and memories with another person, consider yourself lucky—what a privilege to share part of another's journey. No one has to let you be in their life. If we all really looked at being in someone's life as a blessing and a privilege, wouldn't we treat them better and with much more sensitivity? When someone becomes our friend, they open the door to their life and say, "Come into my world." They don't have to let us be there. Recognize that. Thank them for that. Thank them for allowing you to share in their journey. As the poet Javan said, "Touch gently the life of your fellow man. For the human heart shapes as easily as clay upon the potter's wheel."

Wouldn't it be nice if life came with a script telling us all the right things to say at all the right times? Maybe you've thought of giving someone a compliment, but chose not to, when it just may be what was needed to make a difference in that person's life in that moment. Have you ever wondered which hurts most, saying something and wishing you hadn't or not saying anything and wishing you had? Choose your words wisely. Yes, words can be magic, but magic can sometimes be illusion. I'm not suggesting false flattery, which most people can see through immediately, but instead, a greater consciousness toward sharing words of kindness.

As I progressed throughout the entire journey—whether it was the first of hundreds of dieting attempts, exercise attempts, gym memberships, personal trainers, hypnosis, whatever it was—I always focused on the words my mom and Nonnie spoke to me: "I believe in you and you can do this." It is so important to know who is in our corner and who we can count on for support. My mom and Nonnie never once said to me that I couldn't make it, or I should give up, or oh boy, here we go again. They never did anything but support every single effort I ever made. I was also blessed with an amazing best friend, Lori, who also believed in me and supported all of my efforts. She wasn't big at all, but she always tried to understand and help me any way she could. She would listen to me on the phone for hours at night. She never gave up on me either. Truth is, I didn't believe in myself at all. I hoped I could make it, but deep inside I doubted it. But those three women, they believed in me, they championed me, they supported me, and it made a huge difference in my life. They never gave up on me.

Not everyone in my life was supportive, because that's the truth of living. I hope with all I have that as I retell these stories around this planet of ours, many will hear me and will think twice before they say the painful things I have shared here. That is part of my entire mission: Help the hurters to stop hurting and help the hurting to stop hurting. Sadly, so many times the people who hurt us are the ones we love the most. I have spoken to so many hurting people and have found that many, many times those who love us don't realize the impact their hurtful words have on us. They erroneously think that their words will motivate us.

My own father was helping me renovate my new home and we were putting in a large, garden tub because I couldn't fit in a regular sized bath tub very well, at least, not if I wanted water in there, too. The plumber was there with my dad and he said, "Wow, that's a BIG tub!" My dad responded and said, "Well, she's a BIG girl!" I was standing out in the hallway when I heard those words and I just walked quietly outside. I know how much my dad loved me, but he was one of those people who didn't choose words very well. And to make it even worse, he also believed that if I didn't like people saying those things then I should do something to change it. He thought I just didn't work out hard enough and didn't eat right. He was wrong.

As I once heard Dr. Phil say, there are two lines in life. There is the line for "people who get it" and the line for "people who just don't get it." Guess which line my dad was in when it came to my weight? I'll bet some of the people you love stand in the same line. Some people in life will eventually realize that they have been in the wrong line and adjust accordingly. Others will remain stuck in their same line forever. The important thing to remember is that we can't change people or the line in which they are standing. Eventually if we allow our opinions of ourselves to be formed by others' perceptions of us, then aren't we standing in the wrong line as well?

Never give another person the power to make you think less of yourself. As Eleanor Roosevelt said, "No one can make you feel inferior without your consent." Firmly claim the ground beneath your feet, stand in the powerful line of people who get it, and announce to yourself and the world, "I will never allow your perception of me to affect my opinion of me."

Words are powerful. As Edward Thorndike said, "Colors fade, temples crumble, empires fall, but wise words endure." Unfortunately, hurtful words persevere as well. I don't believe there is a statute of limitations in our memory for pain. I do believe, though, that we can choose to channel that pain into something positive. We have to always remember, we are more than our bodies, more than our pasts, and more than any memories we have of how we've been treated. We can't change what we've been through, but we are responsible for how we respond. Choose something better. As Oprah says, "The best revenge is to live well."

Make the powerful choice today to live well. For each and every one of you trying to find your own way to lose weight, whether you have a support system or not, hear me when I say this: I believe in you and you can do this. If I can do it, anyone can do it. I used to lie in bed at night and when I would think about having to lose 243 pounds, I would think I could never do it. It was just too great a number. I would get more overwhelmed and more depressed. But I eventually did it, and I'm here to tell you about a journey I never thought could happen.

So please, please believe that you can do this. You are not too far gone. You are not too big. You are not too old. You are not too heavy. You are not too anything, but worthy of happiness. There are countless ways to find the best way for you. I BELIEVE IN YOU AND YOU CAN DO THIS!

"Sometimes you've got to believe in someone else's belief in you until your own belief kicks in."

—Les Brown

CHAPTER 3

"Imagination is everything. It is the preview of life's coming attractions."

—Albert Einstein

There were many factors, situations, and people who contributed to my eventual decision to have bariatric surgery. It wasn't an immediate decision on my part, and I vacillated many times about whether to actually go through with it or just keep trying to diet and exercise on my own. In fact, I attended an informational session a few years prior to my actual surgery and decided not to go through with it at that time due to financial concerns and the never-ending hope that I could somehow lose the weight without the need for surgical intervention.

My hesitation is one of the things I actually regret. I probably put the surgery off for three or four years, and those were years of my life I could never get back. A prisoner held captive in my own body, I was mired in unhappiness. The surgery actually released me onto a path of becoming a new, healthier, happier person. How different would my life have been if I had the surgery the first time I checked into it? That's a question I'll never know the answer to, but I'm a firm believer that every single thing that happens in this life happens at the perfect time. God is always on time. There is a common saying: "When the mind is ready, a teacher appears."

For whatever reason, it wasn't my time yet. I always did things in my own time and I always believed that there is a way for everyone and there are infinite ways to find your own way. I have to admit, it took me a while to find my way. As much as I desperately wanted to lose the weight, I was also terrified. At the time, I didn't even realize what terrified me. Fear is a powerful opponent and if you allow it, fear will be an adversary you can never defeat. But keep in mind: you can't be a champion without an opponent. My biggest opponent was all of the thoughts and fears in my mind. I now know that in reality, I was actually afraid to lose the weight because then I would have to deal with the reasons I used it as a barrier to insulate and protect myself from others in the first place. At the time, though, if I thought about something long enough I could come up with a million completely irrational thoughts and convince myself they were on target. That's what fear does. Fear had me riding right on top of that float in the Homecoming parade at Crazy Town. I was waving enthusiastically to my supporters and to the people in the crowd. And all of those crazy people were wildly waving back. But remember, we are talking about Crazy Town. It's not a good place to visit, let alone live.

While my own fear kept me immobile, there was also another issue at hand: not everyone supported the idea of surgery. Some friends, family members, and coworkers thought it was ridiculous to have surgery to lose weight, saying I must be lazy or not disciplined enough to lose the weight on my own.

Back then, I allowed that type of thinking and those kinds of negative people to infiltrate my thoughts and affect my decision. I never considered that perhaps those people had their own reasons for not wanting me to be successful in my weight loss. Those friends always said they supported me and that they would do anything to help me in my weight loss, but every time I spoke of surgery they would get upset and speak out against it. Some of them even had weight problems of their own, but when I would discuss the surgery they would say that they would never do something like that.

The implication from my detractors was that I was somehow a sell-out for taking the "easy" way out and having surgery to help in my weight loss. I distinctly remember one person telling me that by having bariatric surgery I would be opening Pandora's Box—I would have a bigger set of problems after the surgery because everyone she knew who had the surgery had major problems. They may have lost some weight, but eventually they gained back even more weight and became a bigger size than they were when they started.

With so many people using the "Pandora's Box" analogy on me, I decided to learn more about the actual myth and give it some thought. I found that so many people speak of the mythical story without knowing the entirety of its message. Pandora was actually created out of clay by Zeus, the most powerful of the mythical Gods. He created her to punish Epimetheus. Epimetheus and his brother, Prometheus, were both Titans with big hearts. When Zeus had punished humans by taking away fire, these brothers, who realized how much humans needed it, felt sorry for them. They then stole the fire back and returned it to them. This enraged Zeus. He chained Prometheus to a rock for many years and then created Pandora as part of his deceptive plan to punish Epimetheus as well. Zeus used the help of the other Gods to make Pandora irresistible to Epimetheus and then sent her as a gift to him. Epimetheus fell in love with Pandora and despite the warnings of his brother to not trust Zeus, he married her quickly. As a wedding present, Zeus presented Pandora with a beautiful box on their wedding. The message he included with the beautiful box told Pandora that she and Epimetheus would always be happy as long as she never opened the box. The two were having a fabulous married life together, but Pandora was always curious as to what was contained in the beautiful box.

When, as Zeus had suspected, curiosity got the best of Pandora, she waited until her husband was out of the room and she, alone, opened the box. Immediately Pandora discovered that the box contained pure misery. Zeus had filled the box with the evils of the world—death, envy, pain, suffering, sadness, disease; all of those were released as flying bugs that swarmed out of the box and began to bite and sting Pandora. Pandora's husband heard her agonizing screams and came and quickly helped her shut the box. They realized though, that they heard a small voice crying to be released from inside the box. Something was trapped. Deciding that nothing more terrible than what had already occurred could be released, Pandora and Epimetheus opened the box and were surprised to find hope cowered in the corner. Whereas the evil had been composed of stinging, flying bugs, hope was likened to a gossamer dragonfly. Hope fluttered around and landed on and healed every wound that the evils had inflicted on Pandora. The box was full of evil, but even still, in the very end, there was hope. It turns out that Zeus, in spite of all of his anger and fury, still had some love for the humans and showed mercy by placing hope in the box as well.

This mythical story became important to me, and I share it now because when I had my surgery there were many changes that came along with it, and not all of them were as easy to navigate as one might think. I have to admit that my friend who likened the surgery to Pandora's Box was right in many ways. The surgery did bring some complications into my life. However, just as with Pandora's box, while there were many new challenges I had to learn to accept, the most beautiful thing in the world, something I had lived without for many years was returned to me, and that was hope.

It is dangerous to grow accustomed to living safely behind your fears and the fears of others. I had allowed all of the weight on my body to serve as a moat to protect my soul; a defense against all hurtful attacks. While the moat worked to some extent in keeping people away from me, it certainly didn't make me feel any better. The moat kept out the hurtful people and some of the hurtful things. But the moat also kept out many of the good people and the good things. Isolation keeps out everything until suddenly you're left alone with your inner negativity, still hearing the assault of stinging from the outside. I certainly wasn't healing and finding happiness inside the castle of my soul. My soul and my heart were secluded. While seclusion can sometimes be helpful, it is not a healthy way to live. At the core was the silent question in my mind that without the weight I still wouldn't be enough—the weight might be a burden but it was, at the very least, a convenient excuse for my pitfalls.

My soul refused to go down quietly, though. It refused to let me wallow for long or to allow me to simply accept myself as being less than I was created to be. My soul had a voice, and that voice was loud and constant. Sometimes that voice was downright annoying. I would constantly have dreams about my weight. When I was in high school, cheerleading was my favorite sport. Once I was heavy, I would have dreams that I was trying out for cheerleading again at my current size. I was panicked and devastated because I wanted so desperately to be a cheerleader and I knew I couldn't at almost 400 pounds.

In my dreams, I would try to tell the judges that I would lose the weight before the season started. I would implore them to give me a chance and even ask my friends to vouch for me. It sounds silly, but I would wake up distraught and then have to tell myself that it was only a dream. I would be so upset when I woke up that I would have to remind myself that I had been a successful cheerleader in high school. I was in my thirties and high school was in my very distant past, but still I couldn't shake the feeling of being inadequate. I had the dream constantly for years, until it became so common that I could refer to it in shorthand to my best friend: "I had the cheerleader dream again." Then she would give me a long sigh and say, "Oh, no." She was a cheerleader with me in high school and knew how passionate I was about it. My time cheering with her are some of my best memories. So, she deeply understood how much these dreams were haunting me.

I experienced that same dream hundreds of times over several years. Sometimes the details of the dream changed based on what was going on in my life. My son's father was a magnificent basketball player. He played high school, college, and professional basketball overseas. Everyone knew who he was and what an incredible athlete he was. In the years that we were together, he would sometimes appear in my dream. Our relationship was in no way perfect, but I knew that he loved me the best he could. In my dreams, he would be in high school with me and he would tell his basketball coaches that if I didn't get to cheer, he wouldn't play basketball. Because of his talent, the coaches would always strong arm the cheerleading advisor and they would put me on the squad so that he would still play basketball for the team.

Isn't it incredible how our psyche and our soul speak to us in ways we can't shut down? My dreams were one of the major factors that pushed me toward the decision to have surgery. They were constantly mirroring my life. My son's father loved me in spite of my weight. Despite our problems, he loved me regardless of the way I was seen by the rest of the world. In my mind, he was capable of looking past all of my weight and still finding something beautiful. He swam right across that moat I thought would keep people away. In his presence, I felt beautiful, protected, and loved. So, of course, he showed up in my dreams in the exact same way he did in my life. We were a package deal. But sometimes our souls know more than we do, and the fears that I had were resounding loudly in my mind without backing down. I couldn't deny their reality just as I couldn't deny the complication that comes from needing support while also needing to strive toward a better life.

Even though my son's father and his supportive presence in my life was a beautiful thing, it still was the kind of support that enabled me to stay less than happy. It supported my feelings of being inadequate in most areas. Just as in the dream, I was nothing if he wasn't beside me. I was just the fat woman who people looked beyond. Who I was dating and involved with made me more acceptable to the rest of the world. That's so sad and embarrassing, but it was my truth. Who was I without him? I was really sitting on my throne at that point. The Homecoming Queen of Crazy Town was in prime form during those years, but despair and unhappiness provide fertile soil for the unthinkable to grow. In spite of the fact that we had a lot of love between us, our relationship was not a healthy one built on respect. I stayed in that relationship longer than I should have because I didn't want to lose him. But more significantly, I didn't want to lose the acceptance I felt from being with him.

People were always surprised when they would meet my son's father. It was as though I were more acceptable in their eyes because I had an attractive, charming man in my life. Sadly though, people were very vocal and would ask, "Why is HE with HER?!" No, they didn't say it to my face, but they said it to others, and it always got back to me. In addition, I always saw it in their eyes the moment they met him. They would say that he must have been with me because I had money or for some reason other than love. Never because of my own worthiness.

My dreams persisted for well over a decade. I would wake up from those dreams feeling that my best days were behind me and that I would never be worthy again—to myself or to others. I felt that my days were hard enough and my life was sad enough as it was. I didn't need dreams to reinforce how terrible I already felt. But that is how our soul speaks to us. I have heard that the soul will not be quiet until what it wants is achieved. My soul could not rest living in a body that was holding me back from what I was meant to become. My soul was persistent, an emotional stalker that harassed me even in my sleep. My soul simply would not stop. It nagged me. But without a doubt, I can say that my soul was heard, eventually. I got its message loud and clear. I just wasn't sure what I was going to do about it.

While this was going on, I would watch daytime talk shows that spotlighted people who had lost significant weight through surgery. They would show a "before" picture of someone, and then that person would walk out on stage looking completely different. These people were thin and healthy and smiling. I would sit on my couch and watch those shows with tears streaming down my face.

What those shows did for me was provide a glimpse of how my life could possibly be transformed. They opened a window that I could gaze into and see options I hadn't considered before, ways to change my current situation. In short, watching those shows gave me hope, and hope was something

I had been without for a long time. I would call my mom to talk about those shows and the surgery that those people had, and I would ask her if she thought it was possible for me, too. My mom had always supported everything I wanted to do, but she wasn't completely certain about the surgery. In addition, my health insurance didn't cover the incredibly expensive surgery and I didn't have the money to pay for it myself.

While simply the weight alone was enough to be a physical and emotional burden, I also began having some very serious health issues. I had to be medicated for both high blood pressure and migraines. Eventually, my eyes really started to bother me and were very, very dry and itchy. I was diagnosed with Floppy Eye Syndrome. The eye doctor I saw asked me if I ever slept with my eyes open and recommended that I check with my partner to find out.

I thought that I certainly didn't have this strange disorder of Floppy Eye Syndrome, because my doctor said that it was most commonly associated with obese people. In spite of weighing almost 400 pounds, I didn't want any illness that was known to be prevalent among the obese. That's how my mind worked at the time. Part of me still lived in denial, and I definitely didn't want to be diagnosed with anything that had a correlation to obesity. I asked the man I was seeing if he ever noticed that I slept with my eyes open. His response stunned me. He said, "Yes, and it's the strangest thing. If it weren't for the fact that you're snoring, I'd swear you're looking right at me. It freaked me out at first, but now I'm used to it." Because I was diagnosed with this strange affliction, I had to begin taping my eyes shut at night to sleep. More alarmingly, however, I found out this syndrome is also usually associated with sleep apnea.

While doing my research on both disorders, I read that sleep apnea could be fatal. I read the list of symptoms and had a sinking feeling in my stomach because I recognized most of them. I shut my computer off and decided to think of something else. At that time, I couldn't deal with the seriousness of what I apparently had. My son was only six when I received this diagnosis, and I couldn't bear to think of not seeing him grow up. It was a pain I couldn't bear, so I set all of my concerns, fears, and symptoms aside on that mental shelf we all have that allows us to live in the dangerous safety of denial.

I thought of the surgery on a daily basis. I would lie awake at night and wonder how different my life might be if I had it. I would daydream before falling asleep about how I would look if I were thin. What would I wear? What man would I date? What could I do when I wasn't held back by my own body? Sometimes it is necessary to daydream in order to move away from dwelling on what is painful. Sometimes, daydreaming can be a way to acknowledge our problems gently and with the kind of hope found in Pandora's Box.

Our minds are our most powerful asset. Without realizing it, for years I was utilizing the Law of Attraction. The

Bible states in Mark 11:24-25, "That which you ask for in prayer and believe, you shall receive." The Law of Attraction is founded from this principle and simply states, "Ask. Believe. Receive." One of the powerful forces of the Law of Attraction is visualization. Without my realizing it, those years of daydreams before bedtime eventually were fulfilled by the Universe and God.

Rather than facing my troubles head on, I could begin to accept their reality by imagining a life without them and believing that it was possible to change. If there is anything to remember in this search for peace in my own body, it is that hope sits right beneath the worst parts of ourselves and our fears, begging to be released. We have the power and the capability to make our dreams come true.

"To accomplish great things we must not only act, but also dream; not only plan, but also believe."

—Anatole France

CHAPTER 4

"Hope itself is like a star—not to be seen in the sunshine of prosperity, and only to be discovered in the night of adversity."

—Charles H. Spurgeon

It's funny how hope works. I can honestly say that sadly, there have been a few times in my life when hope went missing. Those were very dark days and something I sincerely pray I never experience again. There were times when I felt that everything I needed or wanted had either been taken from me or denied to me. I couldn't see past the disappointment of what I truly believed I needed. It appeared as though certain choices were my only option, and when those choices didn't work out, I became filled with despair and hopelessness. I felt like I was standing alone and no matter which way I looked, I couldn't see anything. No matter which way I reached, there was no one and nothing. I felt alone, in the darkness. It was a very dark night of my soul.

But hear me when I say this, there is always, ALWAYS hope. In our darkest of moments, we should always allow faith to float to the top and we should always eventually settle into a place of hope. Hope should never be AWOL, or go missing from our lives. My favorite Bible verse, which has gotten me through many difficult times, is found in Isaiah 22:22: "When He opens doors, no one will be able to close them; when He closes doors, no one will be able to open them." I believe that God opens the doors we need to walk through and He closes the ones that will hurt us or don't have anything we need behind them.

This point is illustrated perfectly in my surgical story. I had finally decided I was going to have the surgery. Despite all of the people who made it blatantly clear that they didn't want me to have the surgery, and in spite of the fact my health insurance wouldn't pay for my surgery, I made the decision anyway. I didn't know how I was going to pay for it, but I decided to worry about that later. I could only slay one giant at a time. Just the ability to say to my friends, family, and the world, "I am having this surgery," was a huge victory for me.

I began to call around and do some research. I had submitted several requests and reports from doctors stating that surgery was a necessity for me, but my insurance refused to budge. Regardless, I continued my march onward to find the right surgeon for me.

I called to schedule my second informational session with Dr. Maguire at Kettering Hospital in Kettering, Ohio. I had attended an informational session with Dr. Maguire several years prior. He was the surgeon that everyone I knew or had spoken to had recommended, and he was my first choice. While there were several different types of bariatric surgery at the time, Dr. Maguire did the type I wanted, the biliopancreatic diversion with the duodenal switch. Not many other surgeons performed that procedure.

The reason I chose this particular procedure is because it was malabsorptive, meaning the patient didn't absorb the calories from everything that was eaten. It was Dr. Maguire's "surgery of choice." In fact, he called it the "Cadillac of bariatric surgery." He stated in the seminar that this surgery had the best long-term results for keeping the weight off permanently. One thing I knew for sure was that if there was a way to gain the weight back, I would find it. I had also researched other surgical procedures and found that some of them had poor percentages of weight regain. The research on one popular version of the surgery at the time stated that within ten years, 100 percent of people had gained back at least 50 percent of the original weight they had lost. I didn't want that to happen to me.

When I made the call to schedule an informational session, I was surprised that I was going to have to wait quite a while to attend one, as they were booked up for a few months. I was very disappointed because I had finally made the decision and didn't want to wait months just to get to this first step. The previous session I had attended did not help me at this point because too much time had elapsed. I cried when I hit this roadblock, and I felt that door was closed to me. I did, however, go ahead and schedule the session that was a few months away and Kim, Dr. Maguire's assistant, told me that she would put my name on the waiting list in case an earlier opening became available.

My impatience got the best of me and I decided to call other surgeons and try to get into one of them. The next surgeon I called was available much sooner, but when I stated that my insurance wouldn't pay for the surgery, I was told that they did not take cash payments. The second door was closed to me. I called the third surgeon on my list and was told the exact same thing. A third door closed. Eventually I called around and had spoken to five other surgeon's offices in the state of Ohio, and all of them told me that either they didn't accept cash payments or their surgeon didn't perform the surgery I preferred. I was distraught. I cried and cried, and then did what I always did when I was hurting and disappointed. I called my mom.

My mom said that maybe I should just accept that I wasn't meant to have the surgery. She knew she couldn't help me pay for the surgery at that time, and she had no idea how I was going to come up with the money. She didn't understand why I was getting emotionally invested in a procedure I couldn't afford. I have to admit that at this point, even I thought perhaps I wasn't meant to have the surgery.

I wondered if I was foolish to think that I could come up

with the money to pay for the surgery. My parents had been wonderful at helping me with anything I ever wanted, but they had begun to focus on "tough love" in an effort to make me more responsible. They felt that at this point in my life I needed to begin paying my own expenses.

My parents knew I worked hard, and although they were always wonderful and generous, they wanted to know that I would be okay on my own one day when they were no longer here. And since my dad didn't think I should have the surgery anyway, I knew there wasn't much of a chance they would help me finance the surgery. Whenever I brought up ideas as to how I could pay for the surgery, my mom would respond by saying, "Don't look at me, because we are not helping you pay for this." This comment always hurt my feelings, because to be honest, I was secretly hoping they would acquiesce and pay for it anyway. I found out, however, that it was the best thing my parents ever did for me. It caused me to become totally self-reliant.

A couple of weeks had passed since I had begun my quest to have the surgery. I still hadn't found another surgeon who performed the surgery and would accept a cash payment. Several doors had been closed to me, and I had not decided what to do. I was devastated.

I thought of all the things that being overweight had made difficult for me to accomplish in life.

I had season tickets to the University of Dayton men's

college basketball team. My seats were close to the floor. My best friend Lori and I were college basketball junkies and loved going to those games. Walking down to my seats was not difficult because it was all downstairs, but walking back up was a different story. Throughout the game, I would not go to the restroom because I couldn't walk up all those steps to get to the restrooms. Following every game, we would wait until everyone had cleared out because it was so hard to climb the steps. I usually wouldn't even make it halfway up before I had to sit down and rest because I was tired and out of breath. Lori would always be very patient and talk to me until I could catch my breath and walk the rest of the way. When we got to the top I would have to grab onto the wall and rest again. I would stand there, gasping for breath, sweat pouring off of me. I hated that. I dreaded those stairs. I was both horrified and angered at the fact that it was so hard for me. I always felt that the few people who were still in the arena stared at me with contempt, or even worse, with pity. It was embarrassing.

Strangely enough, that same arena was soon to be the scene of an incident that would ultimately be one of the most significant factors that contributed to my decision to have surgery. I took my son, who was seven, there to see the circus. As we were making our way down the steps to our seats, I had to sit down for a minute to rest my back. My son was obediently standing beside me, excitement dancing in his eyes at the mere thought of all of the magic he was about to experience within the circus. Then an usher came up to me and asked if I had a ticket for the seat I was sitting in. I showed him my tickets and explained to him that my seats were down close to the floor, but I needed to rest my back and then we would be walking the rest of the way down to our seats.

I'll never forget that man. He looked at me with complete disgust and told me that I had to get up out of that seat because I didn't have a ticket for it. At that point, the arena was still mostly empty. I tended to arrive everywhere early so that I could rest a few times between the parking lot and my seat. I didn't want to miss this event so I had planned accordingly.

There was no good reason for this man to treat me with such disrespect and disdain. I was so embarrassed. I was embarrassed for myself and even more embarrassed that my son heard someone talk to me that way. But my son just looked at me with his big brown eyes and said, "I'll hold your hand Mommy, and that will help." I wonder about that man to this day. What was the payoff for his humiliating me and speaking down to me in such a way? It saddens me to think of the personal demons that must have been haunting him to cause him to treat a young mother and her son in that manner.

We walked down to our seats. I was exhausted. It was so hard for me to even walk a few steps at that point. I was never so happy to see my seat and sit down. My heart was racing, I could barely breathe, and I was sweating profusely. I sat down looking at all of the people around me who could walk without any physical problems. I thought about how difficult my life had become and how even something like walking, which most people take for granted, was painful and almost impossible for me. That realization was something that I found deeply disturbing.

A beautiful distraction, however, was my son and the fact that he was completely in awe of the circus. He was so thrilled to be watching all of the electric energy that exudes from the circus atmosphere. Then he saw the elephants. They were dressed with amazing colorful head pieces and had on saddles that were sparkling and glistening. Each one of them was carrying a load of happy and excited children, all smiling and waving to their parents. He begged me to let him ride an elephant. His excitement was unmistakable.

I knew I couldn't walk any farther. I could see other parents standing and waiting for their children to take a ride. I knew I couldn't stand there and wait that long, and I didn't see any place to sit down. I knew my back would hurt too much and I just couldn't physically do it. I explained to him that I didn't think I could make it. On most occasions, my son would accept when I was unable to do something and would even try to hide his disappointment from me. My son, in his young life, had seen many, many tears shed by his mother. He had been witness to many hurtful and painful times I had experienced because of my weight. He was actually quite protective of me, both physically and emotionally.

On this occasion, though, he wasn't giving up so easily. He told me firmly and confidently that he could do it with me watching from my seat. He very carefully explained exactly the route he would take to get to the elephants. He pointed out where he would wait, in my view, and he gave me a concise explanation of precisely how he would accomplish it safely and on his own. He promised me that he would be careful, and he begged me to please allow him to do it alone, under my watchful supervision. The floor was only a few rows from our seats, and even though it terrified me, I had to admit I was quite impressed with his well-delivered, persuasive argument. I did tell him one stipulation was that he had to get a picture taken for me. Even though it terrified me, I gave him the money for both the ride and the picture and sent him off with my blessing to ride the elephant. He was so excited, he hopped up out of his seat, gave me a big hug and kiss, and with that he was off for the circus experience of a lifetime.

As I watched my son walking down to the awaiting elephants, I was so proud of the little boy he was and of how he had the courage to advocate for himself and explain to me that in spite of my physical limitations, he was brave, responsible, and determined enough to accomplish something he really wanted to do on his own. He bounced down those stairs, stood in line, and paid for his ride all by himself. While patiently waiting in line, he looked up at me regularly, waving with great pride and happiness. Finally, it was his turn. He climbed the ladder, stood up on the platform and crawled up on top of the elephant. He rode that elephant as long as they would allow. As the elephant slowly completed each circle and walked past my seat, he looked up at me with the biggest grin and waved like crazy.

Each and every single time that he waved at me, I waved back as enthusiastically as if it were the first. As I was waving and smiling at him from the crowd, tears literally streamed down my face. I was devastated that I could not do all the things I so desperately wanted to share with him. He was so proud of himself and was such a good little boy, and I was eaten alive with guilt that he deserved a better mom than I could be at the time. He deserved someone who could be active and enjoy his life with him. I knew this child adored me exactly how I was, and I also knew that he knew how much I loved him. I was no longer missing just my life, I was missing his as well.

When the much-anticipated elephant ride was over, my son walked over and I assumed he was getting the picture of his big event. I couldn't see exactly what he was doing and there seemed to be a bit of activity going on where he was. After a few minutes, he emerged with a bag in his hand, smiling from ear to ear. When he arrived next to me, he showed me the picture of him on the elephant and then produced a picture of him with a chimpanzee as well. When he'd gotten off of the elephant, he had a photo taken with the chimp as well. He was quite proud of the little extra picture of him and the chimp.

When we left the arena that day, there was a carnival in the parking lot. He looked over at it and then looked up at me and before I could say a word he said, "I don't really want to go to that carnival because I'm kind of anxious to get home and show Grandma the picture of me and that monkey." I knew he was fibbing to protect my feelings. He wanted to go to that carnival, and he knew I couldn't take him. He knew I could never walk that far and I couldn't be on my feet long enough for him to attend the carnival. The words escape me as to just how badly I felt about the fact that my child had to create excuses simply because I was physically incapable of doing the activities he wanted to do. He was trying to protect my feelings. Although it was a beautiful display of his love for me, I still suffered deeply inside. The sad fact was I wanted him to have a better mom than me. Of course, I would never give my son away, so I knew I had to make a change so that I could be the mother he needed me to be.

I felt so terrible. I had a sadness deep in my soul. This was not the kind of mom I wanted to be. Children are amazing though. He never complained. He never said a word about wishing I was smaller or more capable of doing things. He never whined about all of the fun things he missed out on. He just loved me, plain and simple.

One day, he got into a little trouble at school. He was in the first grade and he had kicked a child. The teacher called me, and I was stunned. It seemed so out of character for him. I asked him why he had kicked the other child, and he gave me a reason that just didn't make sense. Finally, after questioning him further, he came clean. This little boy had called me fat and Alec had defended me. The other boy continued with his insults at recess, and my son kicked him in his shin.

I weighed 391 pounds and my son didn't believe I was fat. He loved me and was defending my honor. I'll never forget the look on his face when he finally told me the story. He was so angry that someone had actually said something mean about his mommy. In his little seven-year-old body, he was doing everything he could to protect me and honor me. It broke my heart into a million pieces that he had to go through things like that because of me. While I was beating myself up for not being all the things I felt I should have been, I was startled by my phone.

It was Kim, Dr. Maguire's assistant, and she told me that if I still wanted to attend the seminar, someone had cancelled, and they had an opening in the next one only a couple of days away. Did I want to attend?! Of course I wanted to attend!!! Kim laughed and I remembered thinking that she genuinely seemed happy for me. I was so excited. As if by magic, an opening had occurred. But I know enough to know that it wasn't magic at all. It was God. God opened the door. Even today, I get goosebumps remembering it.

I needed a support person to attend with me. Since it was during the day, I didn't want to ask my best friend, Lori, to miss work. Knowing that my mom wasn't a fan of the surgery, with more than a little fear in my heart, I called her and asked her to please attend with me as my support person. Hesitantly, she agreed. We went to the seminar. and she was very impressed with Dr. Maguire. She felt that he was the very best surgeon to do the surgery and had a wealth of experience, but she still didn't know how I was going to come up with the money.

Strangely enough, I kept falling asleep throughout the seminar. I tried so hard to stay awake and focus, but I just kept drifting off to sleep. I would find out a few months later, after my actual surgery, that I did, in fact, have sleep apnea. This explained why I was always tired and would fall asleep during the day. Following the seminar that day, while driving home, I started to fall asleep at the wheel and thankfully my mom started yelling at me and I woke up. She was so scared, and even though I didn't admit it at the time, it terrified me as well. What was wrong with me? I drove as part of my work and with my son in the car, too. What if I fell asleep then? We didn't realize at the time how sick I truly was. I didn't know how much my body was going through and how hard it was working simply to survive.

In spite of my drowsiness, the thing I remember most from attending that seminar was my impression of Dr. Maguire and his assistant, Kim. Dr. Maguire had the quiet resolve of a champion. He exuded a strength and confidence that is rare, and yet he had a kindness and a goodness that was unmistakable. He was a man of few words, but his words were significant. It was overwhelming for me to think of all the lives he had changed and ultimately saved. When I had my individual consultation with Dr. Maguire, I told him that one of my doctors had said that I just needed to eat less and exercise more. I'll never forget his response. He said, "I could argue that point with him and I would win." It was so clear to me that Dr. Maguire knew the struggle and pain of an overweight person. I knew that I was in the presence of greatness. It was crucial to my success that I found a surgeon whom I felt safe with and who I felt had the expertise needed to perform my surgery. My soul immediately felt as ease. I knew he was the one. I knew I had to have Dr. Maguire perform my surgery. What I didn't know was how I was going to pay for it. But I knew I was going to figure it out.

Dr. Maguire was amazing. He was everything I needed to captain the team that was going to help me change my life. And his assistant, Kim? She was overwhelming to me. She was like an angel on earth. I'll never forget my first encounter with her. She was so beautiful. She had that beauty that unmistakably pronounced to everyone, "I am just as beautiful on the inside as I am on the outside." She had long blonde hair and green eyes that were filled with kindness. She was so happy and upbeat, and it was almost as if she twinkled when she walked into the room. I can remember looking at her and thinking if only I could be her size and look like her. Usually someone so pretty made me feel insecure because I always felt that they would laugh at me or look down on me for being so big. But the minute I met Kim, I knew my hurting heart was safe in her presence. She seemed to ooze kindness and goodness out of her pores. I don't even know how many patients she saw that day, but she made me feel special—like I mattered and I was the only person she had to see.

The Queen was in rare form that day, and I'm sure I was a maniac. I had so many questions and concerns, and I was afraid of everything. Kim was incredibly patient with me. She never seemed exasperated or annoyed. I have many stories to share about Kim, but one of the most powerful things she ever said to me, she said on that first day. While we were in the exam room I said, "If I could actually make it to my goal weight, I would be so happy, it would change my life." She looked me right in the eye and said with total sincerity, "With this surgery and Dr. Maguire, it's not going to be an IF you reach your goal weight, it's going to be a WHEN you reach your goal weight." She said it with such strength that I knew she wasn't just an angel of kindness and beauty, she was also an angel of strength and conviction.

Kim had an effervescent laughter that filled the room. Her happiness and positivity were so contagious, and she lightened up the rather serious and quiet Dr. Maguire. In a light-hearted way, Dr. Maguire and Kim were like Batman and Robin. He had been blessed with the superpower of the ability to change and even save a life. She was right there, by his side, as his beautiful sidekick, helping him fight the evil force of obesity and the ignorance that surrounds it. This wasn't just a job for either one of them, it was a mission. They both had a rare understanding of the pain that obese people live with every single day, and because of their compassionate nature, they had both made it a career choice to help as many people as possible. They weren't just showing up for a day's work and receiving a paycheck. They both truly believed in their fight against obesity and in the people who were suffering, both emotionally and physically, from the disease.

Dr. Maguire possessed a precise understanding of the fact that when it comes to morbidly obese people, our bodies can actually work against us. He possessed the intelligence that allowed him to grasp that essential scientific fact, a fact to which many other professionals seem to be oblivious. He and Kim worked together every day trying to help other people not only improve their health, but their overall lives. Equally as important, they treated every patient with honor and dignity, regardless of size or age.

In a society in which I was used to being isolated, laughed at, and treated as a second-rate citizen because of my weight, encountering that level of genuine kindness and respect from Dr. Maguire and Kim felt amazing. My heart, which was bruised and hurting, was in desperate need of that pure kindness. These two people, strangers to me before this day, inspired me, and more importantly, believed in the fact that I could make my dream of losing weight a reality. In just one consultation, the hope they instilled in me was strong enough to quiet all of the painful negativity I had been encumbered with for the last fifteen years. Their sincerity, concern, and complete acceptance felt like something I had never experienced. They were both confident and strong in their convictions that every single one of their patients longed for and deserved something better. In their own special and powerful way, they were fighting for the lives of people who had long ago lost their voice. Angels are warriors, too, you know, and on that day, when I left Dr. Maguire and Kim, I knew that I had just encountered two warrior angels.

"Keep away from people who try to belittle your ambition. Small people always do that, but the really great make you feel that you, too, can become great."

—Mark Twain

CHAPTER 5

"When you truly want something and go after it without limiting yourself with disbelief, the Universe will make it happen."

—The Law of Attraction

I WENT HOME that night determined to figure out a way to pay for this surgery. I thought of my life and what it had been like for the last several years. I was so miserable. I was unhappy, and I was trapped in a body in which I just couldn't live my life and be happy. All of the hurtful comments people had said to me over the years were flooding into my mind, and the tears began spilling over until I was sobbing. I was an unhappy person, and my mind was racing with memories of the countless times people, even those who loved me, used my weight against me.

Alec's father and I had split up five years prior when Alec was only a toddler. As much as I knew that man loved me, while we were together, he would use my weight as an excuse for his poor behavior. Even though I knew that at this point it was emotionally counterproductive, I allowed myself to venture back five years, into the history of our time together, mentally retracing the steps of our relationship.

We were young and in our twenties when we first began dating. He was an attractive, professional athlete. He not only had his choice of women, but to say women chased him everywhere would be the understatement of a lifetime. Not only that, they were also willing to do outrageous things vying for and just hoping to obtain his attention. I never did quite understand how he ended up with me. He could have had anyone, and he chose the fat girl. Everyone wondered why he was with me, so of course I didn't think I deserved him.

There were so many times that he made me feel beautiful and made my heart at ease with him. I knew he loved me, and in him I found the acceptance I was starving for. But with the good came the bad. He also used my weight against me, and that was probably one of the most hurtful things I had ever experienced. I couldn't understand someone who, at times, made me feel so wonderful and who obviously loved me so much, being the same person who could cut me so deeply with his words and actions.

If we were arguing, he would throw the word "fat" around to hurt me. As soon as the words left his mouth, I could see the regret on his face. But once cruel words have been given a voice, they can't be silenced in the mind of the intended victim. Every time I looked in the mirror I would replay those comments over and over in my mind. When I was choosing clothes and getting dressed, I heard those words. When I was putting on my makeup and styling my hair, I heard those words. When I went out, I would look at other women who I thought were beautiful, and in comparing myself to them, I would hear those words. I would fall asleep hearing those words. It was as if there was a repeat button in the iPod of my soul that replayed those piercing comments. I desperately needed a new playlist.

I want to make sure to point out that I was not an innocent victim. My intention is not to portray Jeff as the bad guy. I was such an unhappy person at the time, and in retaliation to the hurtful words he would say to me, I would lash out at him as well. His poor behavior didn't give me a right to behave inappropriately as well. My hurt found a way to voice itself, and my words weren't kind either. As I've said before, hurt people, hurt people. I would say hurtful things to him in reaction to his comments, yet he always appeared to have zero reaction to my words.

Jeff was a confident person, and nothing I said ever really appeared to hurt him. He was confident in who he was, and that confidence provided a shield, an invisible protective barrier, that didn't allow my words to penetrate and reach his soul. It was a miraculous force field I envied, and one that I didn't possess at that time. I wanted so desperately to have a protective shield of my own, but I wasn't capable of that kind of self-acceptance and confidence. My protective shield was constructed of 391 pounds of fat that certainly didn't hide me or shield me from anyone.

I'll never forget one of the many instances in which I found out that he had cheated on me. During the argument over that situation, he told me that he loved me, but he could never be faithful to a "big woman." I was crushed. He actually told me that I needed to be a "size six panty." He said that size was "perfect." Those words were etched forever in my heart. If only my memory had a delete trash button like a computer, I would love to erase that comment from my memory. Remembering that comment today only evokes in me an eye-roll coupled with a head-shaking sigh. I will never forget the pain that accompanied that conversation. On second thought, I suppose some pains and heartbreaks are meant to be remembered. As George Santayana said, "Those who cannot remember the past are condemned to repeat it."

But on that particular day, I didn't even know what size panty I wore. I only knew for damn sure I wasn't a size six. I was 391 pounds. Of course, those comments hurt me deeply, and I internalized them. I had also heard from quite a few different people that he would say that when we first started dating I wasn't overweight. According to his version of history, I had gained all of my weight since the beginning of our relationship, and that was why he wasn't faithful to me. Hearing this blatant lie hurt and angered me. I had been a big woman since the day I met him. I didn't understand. How could it be that he was so good to me in private, but then would say and do these things when he was away from me? I arrived at the conclusion that just like everyone else, he was embarrassed by both me and my weight. Not only could he not be faithful to me, but he had to make excuses for why he was involved with me as well.

I will never forget the despair I felt. I had frantically called my mom and when she arrived at my home, I was lying on the floor, my face in the carpet, sobbing hysterically. I can honestly remember thinking I had never felt that kind of pain in my life. My mom, who always knew what to say, simply said, "I'm sorry. You deserve better and you should demand better." As I lay there crying, my mind raced with the ramifications of the information I had just received. I thought he was the one person who loved me as I was, who could make me feel beautiful as a woman, and who was able to see beyond all my imperfections and truly love me, without limitations. But, he wasn't. He was ashamed and embarrassed by me, too. The walls of the not-quite-yet-condemned building that housed my soul came crashing down around me.

I don't believe the words exist that could accurately convey the deep pain and sorrow I felt within this situation and this relationship. As much as I loved him, eventually, that little voice inside me was driving me nuts. You know the voice. We all have one. That voice that won't be silenced; that intuitive force that is the BS filter. Well, my voice was screaming at me from within. Even at 391 pounds, I knew I deserved better. I finally realized that his cheating was not a reflection on my weight or the woman I was, it was a reflection on him and the man he was. Who the hell was he to tell me that he was cheating on me because of my damn panty size!!?? All of the disrespect, the cheating, the lying, and the heartbreak, all of the tears that had eventually cried themselves away, they all flooded the valley of my soul, and it was simply too much. I had finally reached my breaking point.

The floodgates of my heart burst open, and finally my self-respect was released. It was a very small amount of self-respect, and I don't know exactly where it originated from, but I thought to myself that even if no other man alive was ever attracted to me, even if I was alone forever, it was better than living this way. In one glorious moment, I ripped that tiara off of my head and threw it across the room like a quarterback who throws a Hail Mary pass successfully into the end zone. The Homecoming Queen of Crazy Town was dethroned, even if only momentarily, while I embraced a rare, life-changing moment of clarity, self-love, and self-respect. It was an incredibly powerful moment.

On that day, in that moment, I chose myself. It was a decision I would never regret. While I know how much Jeff loved me, the simple truth was that we weren't compatible on all the levels we needed to be. I needed to love myself before I could love anyone in the way they needed to be loved. Learning to love myself and embrace the woman I am was not a quick journey or an easy process. In fact, it is a never-ending journey that I still walk today. Healing is a lifetime event. It is a process to embrace and one on which to constantly improve. As my Nonnie would say, "It's a crockpot thing, not a microwave thing." Nothing great is accomplished suddenly. I don't believe we ever just arrive at the finish line and pronounce our healing work completed. It takes a lifetime of effort. We each heal differently, and we each have to navigate our own direction. Based on those decisions, we arrive ultimately at our eventual destination.

At the point that I was working toward the surgery, it had been five years since Jeff and I had broken up, and I remembered it like it was yesterday. I wish I could say that those were the only hurtful moments I had experienced, but I think those of us who have been on this battlefield of morbid obesity know that almost every single day there is an emotional attack from somewhere. So many of those feelings and memories were the driving force that had led me to where I ultimately was: lying in my bed praying for a way to get the money to pay for this surgery. I needed the surgery. I felt it was the only hope I had to get to a better emotional place, a healthier body, a happier me, and a better life.

I remembered that Kim had given me several names of companies that would provide financing for the surgery. I will never forget calling one bank and applying for an unsecured line of credit. The woman from the bank called me back within 30 minutes and said I was approved for a very high amount. She told me that she had never had an application for an unsecured loan come back with such a high limit. It was surprising because I certainly didn't have stellar credit. I jumped in my car and went straight to the bank to sign the papers and finalize that loan before someone at the bank caught what surely had to have been an error!

With that loan and my credit cards, I had enough available credit to pay for Dr. Maguire's fee and the hospital fee. I didn't have enough, though, to pay for the anesthesiologist's fee, but I didn't care. I called and paid for Dr. Maguire, and I paid for Kettering Hospital, but I couldn't receive a confirmed date for my surgery until I paid that anesthesiologist's bill. I was still $2500 short. I didn't know what to do. I tried everything. I asked for increases on my current credit cards and was denied. I applied for more loans, but was turned down. I prayed and I waited. I knew that God had already opened the door for me in many ways, and I had faith he would open this door as well.

That afternoon, as I was sitting in my living room, my mom came walking in my back door. She came over to me and handed me a check for the $2500 and said that she loved me and she wasn't going to see this door closed to me because I was a few hundred dollars short of my goal. It was a huge moment. I instantly cried. My mom cried and hugged me and she told me that she hoped this would finally be the answer that would give me my life back. I knew my parents didn't really have the extra money to help me. I also knew that neither my mom nor my dad was completely sold on the notion of surgery. So, this meant the world to me in so many ways. Love reveals itself in countless ways and on that day, the money my parents gave me unknowingly bought me the rest of my life.

In the end, my mom had come through for me. I knew she probably had to talk my Dad into it, but in the end, this incredibly independent woman was there for me, as she had been every single time I had tried to lose weight.

Every time except one.

My mom did NOT support me when I was 15 and had taken syrup of ipecac thinking it would let me throw up my meal and all the calories I had just eaten. My friends and I thought it was a wonderful idea and a quick way to lose five pounds before cheering in the next basketball game. It was not. I was so sick and miserable, and my mom was infuriated at me. She discovered me in the bathroom throwing up everywhere and crying uncontrollably. I tried to convince her I had eaten a bad McChicken sandwich, but she was way too smart for that. In addition, the bottle of ipecac sitting on the counter gave me away. As usual, she shook her head, and walked away, mumbling something about Jesus, Mary, and Joseph.

When I emerged from the bathroom and walked miserably into the kitchen, Mom was on the phone with my

Nonnie cackling and laughing about my current self-induced situation. She made some crack about how deadly those McChicken sandwiches were, and I heard her and my Nonnie snorting and chuckling. My mom and my Nonnie were the perfect partners in crime, pulling me right into their partnership as I grew up, making us a trio. I knew those strong women loved me, and I knew they would move the earth for me, but I also knew they would torture me relentlessly about the deadly ipecac incident.

So with the gift from my parents, I was able to pay for the anesthesiologist. Kim had told me that I needed to have a psychological evaluation before I could have the surgery, as well. I had six months before the date of my surgery, but I decided to go ahead and get it over with as soon as possible. I went to the appointment, a simple interview that lasted about two hours and involved some personality exams. It was clear to me during the course of the interview that the psychologist needed to know that I had a strong support system that could help me cope with the difficult times in my life. This was imperative since up until this point, I had clearly used food to comfort myself and self-medicate through stressful times.

After this surgery, my stomach would be so small I would no longer be able to use food as comfort. Because of this, I believe the psychologist was looking for evidence that supported that I would be mentally strong enough and capable to deal with the changes that would undoubtedly take place in my life. At the time, I thought this evaluation was a joke and didn't place the significance on it that I now can see, looking back. I didn't understand fully that positive changes can also evoke some very stressful and negative outcomes, and a person needs to be able to handle those situations effectively, with supportive people who they can rely on. The doctor told me that he would have my results to Dr. Maguire by the end of the week. I explained to him that there was no hurry because my surgery wouldn't take place for another six months.

These six months seemed so far away to me. I remember thinking to myself that in six months I could have lost a lot of weight on my own. It seemed so unfair I had to wait so long. Dr. Maguire was in high demand, though, and at least I knew that my surgery date was coming, and that my life would be changing soon. Kim had also put my name on the waiting list, but warned me that people rarely cancelled or rescheduled this surgery because it was so important to each one. It was also a lengthy process to get approved for the surgery, so most people clung to their scheduled surgery date like a winning Powerball ticket.

I was still happy though, because I was finally on the right track. Not only did I have a date for the exact version of the surgery I desired, with the exact surgeon I wanted, but it was all paid for. The paperwork was completed, and since I was unhindered by insurance, excessive documentation and approvals were not necessary. All I had to do was wait.

However, being the impatient person I am, waiting was the hard part. I very clearly remember talking with my mom only a week after I had completed the last required item on the pre-surgery checklist. It seemed that I had been waiting forever already. I didn't think I would ever be able to make it through the next five months and three weeks.

Meanwhile, the comments from friends and family still continued. Just like the people themselves, some were positive, some were negative, and some were ambivalent. I am quite certain that I was on the path to driving them all crazy, especially those special people who comprised my inner circle.

My inner circle of family and friends was made up of a few rare people in my life who had ridden the roller coaster of my weight issues with me since I was in my early teens. My parents, my Nonnie, and my best friend, Lori, had always believed in me. My son, Alec, had an unwavering belief in me and truly believed that I could accomplish anything in the world. Looking into his big, beautiful, brown eyes gave me all the motivation in the world to change my life. Even though his father and I were no longer together, he supported me as well. Our relationship didn't work out, but love was never our problem. He wanted the best for me and had promised me that he would be there to help take care of me and our son while I was recovering from surgery.

There were some other friends and family who supported me, but their support resembled them, and they drifted randomly in and out of my life. We all have those. They come and they go, but when it comes to being on our team, they aren't first string or even second string. They are more like the scrimmage team. Yet, they all have had their place in our lives, and they serve their purpose. I am thankful for all the people who were in my life. I have learned many lessons from each of them. Some of the lessons were painful and some were joyful, but I wouldn't change any of them because each one taught me something different.

Regardless of how large or small the role they played in my life at one point or another, nearly everyone who knew me had lived through the diets that didn't work for me, the workout ideas that didn't help me, the clothes that didn't fit me, and the emotional outbursts that accompanied these situations. Ultimately, they had supported and loved a girl who wasn't happy. They had personally witnessed the Kelley they had all known and loved be buried under 391 pounds of fat. Her eyes were still the same, but they didn't twinkle as they once did. This Kelley didn't bounce in with love and energy, full of laughs and smiles like the Kelley they had known in high school and college. In fact, this Kelley had trouble walking at all and was always hot, sweaty, and short of breath. This Kelley had to rest and recover just from walking into the house from the front porch. This Kelley wasn't happy, not on any level. But those brave, loyal souls, they strapped into their seats on my emotional roller coaster life, and they rode and they rode with me. They chugged up every hill, raced down the slopes, and survived the loops and turns that life threw at me. More importantly, they loved me, and that love was about to become very important in my life.

Not a week later after lamenting to my mom about the interminable wait, I was lying in my bed watching television when I heard my phone ring. It was Kim from Dr. Maguire's office saying one of their patients had cancelled their surgery at the last moment, and Dr. Maguire had an opening in two weeks. She said she had called me right away because the people ahead of me on the waiting list were all covered by insurance, meaning their paperwork was not yet complete. All of my requirements were finished. If I were willing to take this last-minute appointment, I would need to go to have all of my pre-op blood work done in the next day or two in order for Dr. Maguire to have all the results he needed before completing my surgery.

I've mentioned before that Kim was an angel to me, but she also had the uncanny knack of making phone calls that changed my life. I was so happy, I cried. My surgery was supposed to be taking place in 5 months and 2 weeks, and instead it was taking place in 14 days. Kim said to me, "I am so happy for you, Kelley. I know how much this means to you." I hung up and walked as fast as I could walk next door to my parent's house. I couldn't wait to share this news with them. My mom was thrilled for me and hugged me tight. I went home to call Lori. It was a happy day. All I could think about was the fact that I was NOT going to be huge forever. I was finally going to lose the weight.

I kept remembering Kim's words to me during my initial consultation. "It's not an **if** I make my goal weight, it's a **when** I make my goal weight." I fell asleep that night dreaming of the clothes I would wear when I was smaller and how much better I would look and feel. I was so excited. I couldn't even be mad at nosy Pandora, who unleashed all those evils into the world, because lastly, she released hope, and for the first time in almost a decade, I had some. I had my inner circle who loved me. I had a beautiful little boy who made my life worth living. I had God. I had everything I needed.

The next day I went to do my pre-op blood work and tests and was amazed at how many tubes of blood they needed from me. The nurse taking the blood told me that Dr. Maguire was an amazing surgeon and that he was very thorough. I had to sign forms to have an HIV test, which surprised me. I became fixated on that test. Fear does that. Fear pushes you to focus on some mundane detail, so that the major, anxiety-producing issue can be avoided. There was a side of me that was terrified to have the surgery. I tried not to think about it and didn't verbalize it to anyone, but it was there, hovering just beneath the surface, daring me to chicken out.

Although I have to give fear it's due, being tested for a life-threatening disease was also unchartered territory for me. It was one of those things that you never even consider in your life until you are presented with it. I remembered that my friends had told me that when they applied for life insurance they had to take a similar test and they said in those few days until they received their results they worried themselves sick, even though they had no real reason to be concerned. Suddenly, I felt the same way. What if I was one of those rare people who found out they have some terrible disease when they complete some random medical test?

When I went into my appointment with Dr. Maguire, I asked Kim about the bloodwork and all the tests. I asked how long it took to receive the results of the HIV test. I told her I didn't know why it scared me, but I would be relieved when it came back negative. I don't know why I was so concerned. It wasn't like I was having all kinds of sex. It wasn't like I was having any sex at all. Believe it or not, in spite of my "pretty face," men were not lining up to date me or have sex with me. Although I'm sure I could have dated if I had wanted to, I was too unhappy with myself. Even though I craved companionship and love, I didn't allow anyone to get close to me. I was starving for love, but I pushed it away with everything I had.

Have I mentioned before how wonderful and patient Kim is? She assured me that the HIV test always surprises people and most people respond in the exact same way I did. This beautiful woman was given an inordinate amount of patience. She invited me to call to check on my results if I hadn't heard back from her first.

I called her every single day. I called her twice every single day. I called her in the morning and in the afternoon. She always laughed and said that she didn't have them back yet. I would ask her if that was normal. I would ask if the length of time it was taking was indicative of whether it was positive or negative. She always maintained that gentle, reassuring voice and told me that it was typical and not to worry. At some point she must have hung up the phone and thought to herself that she did not reside in Crazy Town and definitely did NOT vote for me to be Homecoming Queen.

From the beginning, I had told Kim and Dr. Maguire that I was planning on writing about my surgery and weight-loss journey. I told them I was keeping notes about every step of the process. When I would call and check on my results, I told Kim that I would make sure to include this subject in my book. One day when I had called her yet again to check for results, she jokingly told me that I'd better dedicate my book to her! She never became impatient with me, and she always took the time to try to reassure me that everything would be fine.

Finally, after what seemed like forever, my phone rang. It was Kim. She told me that the results of my HIV test were back and that they were negative. She told me that the second she read the results she made sure to call me so that I could finally relax. I was so relieved. Kim just laughed and said, "I told you that you would be fine."

I don't think there are very many people on this planet

who could have the level of patience and true empathy that Kim possesses. She somehow seemed to genuinely understand how I felt even though she didn't struggle with her own weight. Kim was perfect in my eyes. She was the perfect size, and I would have traded places with her in an instant. I couldn't help thinking that maybe one day, with the help of the surgery, I could possibly look as nice as Kim. She was a gift to me. God had guided me to the exact place I was meant to be, with exactly the right people providing my care. God opened the door I needed, and I am so happy, thankful, and blessed that Kim and Dr. Maguire were on the other side.

At this point, my surgery was only a few days away and I was having lunch with a friend of mine. I confessed to her that I was a little afraid. What if it didn't work out? What if I had problems? I had read on the Internet that some people had died during the surgery. I had a little boy, and in spite of having a deep faith in God, I was still scared. I wanted to see him grow up and I didn't want someone else raising him. I hadn't voiced these fears to anyone and it was a little surprising that I was telling this truth to this particular friend. She hadn't been a regular figure in my life, and she had only recently become somewhat close to me. At the time, I wasn't sure why I was sharing this fear with her, but in hindsight I know it was because God chose her to be the messenger carrying a crucial sentiment that I desperately needed to hear.

She said to me that God had opened every door I needed

along the way. She reminded me that after I had researched many surgeons, God had led me right back to Dr. Maguire, who was the expert and the surgeon I so desperately wanted in the first place. God had opened the door for an unbelievable amount of financing to be approved for me when I didn't have the credit score to obtain it, and God had moved my parents to pay for my anesthesia. She reminded me of all the obstacles and stumbling blocks that seemed insurmountable at times, and that God had removed them, one by one, allowing everything that needed to happen to occur so that I could have the surgery. She looked me right in the eye and said that God wouldn't have opened all those doors just to let me die on the operating table. It was a powerful moment and one that I will never forget.

I had everything planned for my surgery. My mom and Alec were going to take me to the hospital. We had to be there at 5:00 a.m. for my 7:00 a.m. surgery. A friend of mine was also going to be there, and she was going to stay until I was in recovery and then take Alec home with her and keep him until I was released five days later. At that point, Alec's father was coming to stay during the week to take care of both me and Alec. Alec was only seven years old at the time and was still on summer break after having completed first grade. My parents lived next door, and they would take care of me on the weekends. We had thought of everything, and we were prepared. One thing was certain, the words my friend spoke to me over lunch, kept running through my mind: "God didn't open all those doors for you so you could die on the operating table."

On the night before my surgery I was so excited, I could barely sleep. As most people do with their best friends, for years I had spoken to Lori every single day. But lately I had really been calling her a lot. I would call her several times a day in those last few days before the surgery. I was bursting with energy and thoughts and needed to go over every single one of them with her. Lori was always there for me. She was always willing to listen and to dissect every single thought and concern I was experiencing. I would have been lost without her. There are some souls we are meant to connect with in a lifetime. She was and still is mine.

I went to bed that night and prayed and thanked God for allowing this surgery to happen. I asked Him to be with me and to calm my anxieties and surround me with the peace that only He can provide. I asked Him to guide Dr. Maguire and to please let me survive my surgery and be able to raise my son and see him grow up. In the quiet of that night, God was there. I fell asleep with the hope of a new existence in my heart.

"Do not be afraid. I am with you."

—Isaiah 43:5

CHAPTER 6

"When he opens doors, no one will be able to close them; when he closes doors, no one will be able to open them.

—ISAIAH 22:22

THERE WAS A flurry of activity in the hospital as the nurses were preparing me for surgery. They started my IV, asked me numerous questions, and quite honestly were like kind angels fluttering around me. It was as if they could sense both my fear and my excitement. I was so excited, but nervous at the same time. They kept reassuring me that I was in the best of hands with Dr. Maguire, and I had nothing to worry about. My mom and Alec were there beside me, telling me that I would be fine. Dr. Maguire had come in, checked on me, and told me that my surgery would last approximately two and a half hours, and then had disappeared to prepare.

The nurses eventually came to take me back to the operating room, and my mom and Alec hugged me, kissed me, told me that they loved me, that they would be waiting on me, and that they would see me when I was out of the recovery room. At the time, I remember feeling those little arms of Alec's around my neck. I said a silent prayer to God begging him to let my surgery go well so that I could look into those beautiful eyes again. As the nurses pushed me down the hall, tears started to stream down my face. One of the nurses noticed, patted my shoulder and told me that I would be just fine. I lay there and looked up into her kind face. It's funny how a moment of gentle compassion can leave a lifetime impression.

There were more people in the operating room than I expected. I had never had major surgery before, and I was surprised at the number of people involved. Dr. Maguire came over to my side and asked me how I was feeling. I looked up at his face and I saw the confident eyes of a man who had completed this surgery countless times. But more than anything, I saw eyes that recognized both the hope and the fear in my own eyes. I had learned that Dr. Maguire could be a man of few words. He didn't engage in a lot of useless, small talk. When he spoke, people listened, and his words were impactful. The last thing I remember him saying to me that morning, before I went under anesthesia, was simple, yet incredibly powerful. (I also have to say that surely no one, even Dr. Maguire himself, realized exactly how prophetic his statement was.) He looked at me and said, "I'm going to take good care of you, Kelley."

The next thing I knew, I was being pushed down the hall with several people pushing machines beside my bed. Alec came running down the hall toward my bed yelling, "Mommy !!!!" He tried to throw his little leg up over my calf and climb up into the bed with me, but everyone immediately started admonishing him to stay off of the bed. My mom grabbed his hand and pulled him back to her. I heard her explaining that he couldn't get up in the bed with me because of all the machines and hoses. He was wearing his little blue sweats that had faux green patches on the knees.

What I didn't realize at the time is that I had stopped breathing in the recovery room, and I was on life support. Machines were keeping me alive. I could only breathe with the help of a ventilator. I have never understood exactly how I knew what Alec had done when he saw me being pushed into the intensive care unit that night, but it was as clear to me as anything that happened. I was somehow watching it all unfold. I could see everything and I could hear everything. Several weeks later, when I described these events to those who were present, they were astonished at my accurate and precise depiction.

I only have a few memories of my time on life support, but the memories I do have are crystal clear and as vivid today as they were then. I was very, very hot. The nurses turned the air conditioning as cold as it would go and because I was still unbearably hot, they brought in two large fans and turned them both on high to blow directly onto me. But I was still hot. My thin, little mom was sitting next to my bed freezing. She was trying to stay warm, and the nurses kept bringing her heated blankets to wrap herself in.

I know that the rules for intensive care dictate that only immediate family could visit, but at one point, I looked up and saw my best friend, Lori, standing at the foot of my bed smiling. When she realized I was looking at her and we were having silent eye contact, she proudly stated, "I'm your sister. They weren't keeping me out." That is my definition of a best friend: someone who will lie, cheat, and break every single rule in order to get close to you and make sure you are okay. Lori, who had always been one of the most honest people I knew, was quite proud of her trickery, and I loved her for it.

Lori wasn't the only one lying her way into visiting me. Jeff, my son's father, strolled into the intensive care unit with a huge smile on his face. He was exceptionally proud of his accomplishment. My mom, who was sitting next to me, got up and gave him a hug. I still had tubes down my throat breathing for me and couldn't speak. My mom asked him how he was able to get in to see me. He said, "I told them I was her husband."

To understand the ironic humor in this, you have to understand that first, Jeff and I were never married, and second, if someone even mentioned the word marriage around Jeff, he would leave with skid marks trailing behind him. Also, my hospital paperwork clearly indicated that I was single. My mom pointed this out to Jeff, and he explained that when he told the nurse he was my husband she had informed him of this fact. She then asked him, again, what was his relationship to me. He said that he looked her right in the eye and said again, "I'm her husband." He said that the nurse told him that if he was willing to lie that blatantly to her face, that he must really want to get in to see me, so she let him in. She did, however, accompany him to make sure he was welcome in my room.

He told me that in spite of everything that had happened between us, he loved me and that his world would never be right if anything happened to me. He told me to get well and that he would be waiting at the house to take care of Alec and me when I came home. It meant the world to me that he came. I knew how much he hated hospitals, and I also knew that he must have certainly had a full-blown panic attack when he had to say he was my husband. To me, that was love in action.

Lying in that intensive care unit on life support, I was faced with the realization that there are all kinds of love in the world. Love has countless faces and stories. It has both started and ended wars, and has proven to be the one entity that remains an enigma. Love blossoms in the improbable and blooms in the uncertain. You just can't underestimate love. Love shines through the darkness and warms the coldest night. Love can be as unpredictable as the weather, but you can never rule love out. It will surprise you every time. Love can be for a second, a moment, a season, or a lifetime. Not every kind of love works out forever, but that doesn't lessen its power or its beauty.

Later that same evening, I woke to the sound of a man sobbing. I drifted in and out of consciousness, and it took me a few minutes to realize that someone was sitting on the foot of my bed. After I focused my eyes as best I could, I realized it was my Dad. He had on a baseball hat, hung his head downward, and rubbed his face with his hand. His shoulders shook as he cried and cried. This was all very unusual for him. He was a man's man, a truck driver, and a very rugged person. I don't think I had ever seen him cry. Ever. I couldn't speak because of the tube down my throat, so I just reached for his hand. He told me that he was so sorry. He said he didn't realize I was so sick and that my body was working against me. He told me he should have offered to pay for my surgery years ago.

In that moment, my heart broke for him. He was such a hardworking, honest man. He was actually my stepfather and had married my mom a few years after my biological father had passed away. But he raised me since I was a little girl, and to me he was a father. He had such a keen sense of right and wrong, and it was so obvious that he was very upset at the sight of his daughter, in intensive care, with machines keeping her alive because she couldn't breathe on her own. He just kept crying and saying that he didn't realize how sick I was. He said over and over that he was wrong and he was so sorry. All I could do was hold his hand. I realized in that moment that every single one of those tears he was crying was filled with love. People express love differently. It's not easy for everyone, and sometimes it's even harder for people to express regret.

I knew what he was thinking. I sensed in him that he was remembering the comments he'd made about my not trying hard enough to lose weight or about my eating too much or being too lazy. He very rarely said those things, but once in a while he did, and I knew he was torturing himself with guilt for ever uttering those ill-conceived words. His emotions were genuine and sincere, and the more he cried, the more I loved him. He finally stood up, kissed me on the cheek, and said he loved me. He told me I was going to be all right. He said that I had way too much of my mother and grandmother in me to not be okay.

The friend whom I had lunch with before my surgery, who had given me that final burst of inspiration, visited me as well. I'm not sure what story she told to gain access to my room, but I woke up and she was there. On this day, I was filled with anxiety. I still couldn't communicate with anyone because of the tube, and I was scared, in pain, and beginning to panic. I was distressed and emotional. I was trying to ask for something and no one could understand what I wanted or needed. Two nurses came in, and with my friend they were trying to figure out what I was trying to ask them to do. They couldn't understand my motions and small gestures, and finally a nurse brought me a pen with some paper. I didn't even have the energy to write, but I scribbled one word on the pad. The word was dad.

My friend right away started saying that my dad was at work and was fine. I was shaking my head emphatically trying to tell her I wasn't asking about my dad. The nurses kept guessing as to what I meant, and I kept shaking my head. I finally started pointing to the ceiling. My friend stared at me, watching me intently as I continued to point at the ceiling. Finally, she stated loudly and with conviction, "She means God !!!!" I started nodding my head yes. Yes, yes, yes!!! My friend knew immediately that I wanted them all to pray with me. She asked me if I wanted them to say the Lord's prayer, and I nodded again. It was such a beautiful moment. Without a second thought, instinctively, both nurses grabbed hands with me and my friend. Forming a circle, all three of them said the Lord's prayer, word for word. The best I could do was follow along in my mind. I immediately fell into sleep.

Months later, my friend would recall the sheer magic of that moment. She stated that a peace came over me immediately and that I was able to relax and instantly go to sleep. There are so many people in the world who don't know the Lord's prayer. I'm sure there are many nurses who don't know the Lord's prayer. But on that day, in that hospital room in Kettering, Ohio, it was not by coincidence that the two ICU nurses who were providing my care knew every single word. God sent them. He knew how much I needed them. They held my hand and shared true, sincere faith with me. I wish I knew their names, because to this day, I would love to hug them, thank them, and let them know what a difference they made in my life.

My mom and those around me eventually told me the entire story of my ordeal. My mom said that when she was waiting for me to come out of surgery, she started to worry when it was taking longer than Dr. Maguire had said it would. Initially she wasn't concerned, but as it got longer and longer, her worries began to increase. She had asked at the desk, but was told they didn't have any information yet. Eventually someone told her that I was in recovery, but that I was having some problems breathing, and they were working very diligently on getting my breathing stabilized.

They waited and they waited. After what seemed like forever to them, Dr. Maguire finally came out and spoke with her and explained to her that he had encountered some major complications in my surgery, but that he had been able to complete it. Once I was in the recovery room and they removed the breathing tube that was inserted for surgery, I had quit breathing. He stated I was on a ventilator and that once he felt I was stabilized enough to be moved, they would take me to intensive care. Hours passed. The person who was waiting to take Alec home had thought they would be out of the hospital by noon, and it was after 9:00 p.m. Alec wasn't budging. He didn't want to leave the hospital until he had a chance to see his mommy.

Around 10:00 p.m., my mom and Alec were informed that I would be moved to intensive care in the next 10 or 15 minutes. They went there to await my arrival. When she saw them wheeling me down the hallway, she said she knew immediately how grave my situation was. Having gone to nursing school, my mom recognized right away that the machines were the only thing at that point keeping her daughter alive. She said that was when Alec saw me, and took off running to climb into the bed with me.

Years later, my mom still became quite upset when she recalled that moment. The nurses had tried to prepare her for what was coming, but it was still incredibly overwhelming for her. One of the nurses told her that she should prepare herself in case I did not live through the night.

My friend, standing nearby, also heard that comment. She grabbed Alec, and they left. Thankfully, he had not been present for that conversation. She loaded Alec in her car, and she cried for the entire 45-minute drive back to her house. All she could do was look in her rearview mirror at the sweet little boy sitting in the back seat, horrified at the thought that she might have to tell him that his mommy died.

When they arrived at her home, she took him inside, and

he instantly began playing with her children. She went outside and was walking around the large pond in her back yard. She said that she must have walked around it a hundred times. She was sobbing and very, very angry at me for having the surgery. She said that she was terrified that I was going to die and that she wasn't going to know how to live with that. All night long she was in fear that her phone was going to ring with news that I had died. She kept my son all week for me, and she recounted how every single day she lived in fear that the worst news was coming. Luckily, that was a call that never came.

My mom, however, was a woman with a different mindset. She wasn't going to entertain the thought of her daughter not living through the night. She told the nurse that I was a fighter and a survivor, and that I would be fine. She had faith in Dr. Maguire and that I was receiving the best care possible. She also had a little discussion with me that night. She told me that not only was I going to survive, but that I was going to be better than I'd ever been. I was going to heal and this would be behind us soon. She said that in spite of my being the baby of the family and the only girl, I was always the strongest of all her children. She told me to fight, to fight harder than I'd ever fought. She reminded me that I had a precious little boy waiting for his mommy to come home. And finally, she told me that God wasn't finished with me yet. He had many, many plans for me and, yes, I would leave this earth one day, but it wouldn't be anytime soon.

I survived through the first night and the nurses continued to tell my family that my condition was very critical and that we had to take things one day at a time. They were not optimistic, as they still weren't certain I would survive. After a few days, though, the outlook became a little more positive. They eventually removed the ventilator, moved me out of intensive care, and into a regular room. I wasn't in that room long at all when alarms started going off and I don't remember exactly what happened, but the next thing I knew I was being rushed down the hall in my bed, with several nurses running and pushing me as fast as they could back to the intensive care unit. Upon my arrival, I was reunited with my old friend, the ventilator. I remember it well, and inserting it is not a pleasant procedure.

My body was still not quite strong enough to breathe on its own yet. This was a small setback, but not a devastating one. I was slowly getting better, but healing takes time. After spending a total of about 3 days on the ventilator, I was again moved to a regular room, and I would remain there for the next few days until I was discharged. I had a roommate and I'm sure she didn't realize that she just had the Homecoming Queen of Crazy Town moved into her room. Since I had left my tiara and sash at home, I'm sure she thought I was just plain nuts. I had ramped up to a whole new level of crazy at this point. Suffice it to say, pain meds are not my friend. To be completely honest, I am a lunatic on pain meds. I was slipping in and out of reality, I wasn't sure where I was all of the time, and I couldn't figure out whose house I was in.

I had a very hard time getting out of bed and walking. My stomach had stitches, staples, and some type of plastic pieces with wires that were keeping my incision together. I had a feeding tube in my stomach, IVs, a Peripherally Inserted Central Catheter, or PICC line, in one arm, and several other monitoring devices hooked up to my body. I can't even begin to explain everything that was hooked up to me, much less its purpose.

An initial aftereffect of the surgery is diarrhea. At one point, because I couldn't get out of the bed quickly enough to get to the bathroom, I had an accident. Obviously, even in my drugged state, I was quite upset about this. We called for assistance, and my mom was trying to help me make it to the bathroom. When the nurse walked into the room, I looked at her and I asked her, "Do you live here? Is this your house?" She looked a little stunned and glanced at my mom who told her I was a crazy person on pain meds. She laughed and said that I seemed so genuine and sincere in my query. Apparently in my drug-induced world, I found this somewhat frustrating. I was determined to find out who lived in this house where I was trapped. I looked at my roommate and said, "Ohhhhh, so this is YOUR house? Well I just pooped in your bed. But, I didn't get it on the comforter and don't worry, we will clean it up." Completely confused, this unfortunate, innocent stranger just looked at me and said, "Ok."

At one point, I thought the nurses didn't like me. I was

certain they were trying to scare me by standing outside my door and hissing to make me think there were snakes in my room. Regardless of who visited me, I would tell them that the nurses didn't like me and that they were hissing outside my door. I can only imagine how that must have sounded. My friends and family, bewildered and somewhat amused, would try to tell me that wasn't the case. I would insist. I literally shared this theory with everyone who walked in my room.

My best friend, Lori, finally, in exasperation, went and looked outside my door and said, "There is NO ONE out here !!!" Immediately, my eyes got big when I heard the hissing again. I told her, "SSSsshhhhhh!!!!!! Listen!!! SEE!!! There it is! They're doing it RIGHT now!!! Where are they hiding??" It was then that she figured it out. The compression devices that were attached to my legs to prevent blood clots would make a hissing sound when they deflated and released air. This happened every few minutes. Every time I heard that sound, I had been completely certain that the nurses-culprits were responsible.

My nurse paranoia continued. One night, at midnight, I somehow got to the phone in my room and called Lori and told her that the nurses were holding me against my will, mis-treating me, and that I needed her to come and break me out of whoever's house I was being held in. I told her it had to be her. She was the only one I trusted and the only one I knew would take care of me. Poor Lori. Bless her heart. She listened to my entire crazy story and then, as any best friend would do, she told me that she was on her way to break me out and that she would be there soon. She hung up the phone, rolled over, and she went back to sleep. She knew my crazy self would forget that phone call in one minute and be onto the next outrageous thing. As long as there were narcotics lessening my pain, there was no shortage of outlandish thoughts ripping through my mind at light speed. The funny thing is that I still remember that phone call.

On my last night in the hospital, I continued to have irrational thoughts and wild dreams. When I woke the next morning, a well-dressed, serious man was sitting in the chair next to my bed. I stared at him for a few seconds waiting for recognition to register in my mind, but it never did. He realized I was awake and said to me, "Well, young lady, you've certainly given a lot of people at this hospital several sleepless nights." I had no idea who this man was and why he was losing sleep over me. I couldn't help thinking to myself, "You think you've had a couple of bad days? You should hear what I've been through. At least no one has held you captive in some strange house you don't recognize." Rather quickly though, I grasped what little focus I was capable of and looked at him intently.

He then introduced himself as Richard Gregg, the Director of Critical Care at Kettering Hospital. For some reason at that moment, his words struck me in such an emotional way. I really wasn't cognizant of how ill I had been or of how many people were worrying and praying for me. Even through the haze of all the pain meds, I was aware of the fact that this man, in charge of an entire division of the hospital, had lost sleep over me, a person he didn't even know. I was very touched by his kindness and sincerity.

Dr. Gregg told me that even though I had paid cash for my surgery, the hospital had submitted my bill to my insurance. Due to the severity of my complications, he felt that my insurance should cover the entire bill. Unfortunately, the insurance company did not feel the same way. They had initially declined to pay because they didn't cover bariatric surgery. They considered my complications, at the time, a result of a procedure they didn't cover, and quite simply, they were refusing to pay for anything. He implored me to file an appeal. He told me to get supporting documentation from all of the specialists who had and would be treating me. Then he said that he, too, would write a detailed letter for me to submit with my appeal.

Because I was a self-pay patient, the fee I paid only covered my hospital stay and all the care necessary for a specific number of days. Those days had almost elapsed, and Dr. Maguire didn't want me to accrue an enormous bill. As a result, they decided to discharge me on the last paid day. The hospital staff called and arranged for numerous medical items to be delivered to my house. The head nurse made certain that those items were there before I left the hospital. If Dr. Maguire had his preference, I would have remained in the hospital for several more days, but he couldn't control my insurance company, so he did everything he could do to assist me. He discharged me as late as he could that evening. I believe I left the hospital at 11:55 pm.

When I went in to the office to see Dr. Maguire for my first post-op checkup, I still had the feeding tube in my stomach, as well as all of my staples, stitches, and clips holding my stomach together, and the PICC line that went into my shoulder/neck. I wasn't feeling the best and was still in a significant amount of pain. It was still so hard to move and walk. I was on oxygen and had to drag the bottle everywhere I went as well. Dr. Maguire had to remove all of those items from my body. He told me that removing the staples might pinch a little bit. Usually those types of things were very difficult for me, but on that day, my mind was stuck on what Dr. Maguire said to me when he first walked into the room.

True to form, Dr. Maguire was a man of few words. He came into my exam room and simply asked me how I was feeling and how I had been. I don't even recall what my response was, but I remember clearly what he said to me. He began by telling me that I had given them all quite a scare and that, at a certain point, they had thought they were losing me. He then told me that when he cut me open to perform the surgery, he discovered that I had a compartmental syndrome. Still to this day I do not completely understand what that means exactly, but it was what he said next that I will never forget.

He told me that when he opened me up and saw my internal complications and condition, he instructed the staff assisting him to sew me back up because he didn't feel that I would survive the surgery. He then turned to walk out of the operating room and was going to give my mom the news. But he said that as he got to the doors to walk out of the room, a power greater than him turned him around and told him that he had to at least try. He walked back in, told the staff to wait, and said he was going to try to complete the surgery because I wasn't going to live much longer without it. And that is what he did.

He told me that while in the recovery room I was stable until they removed the surgical breathing tube. That was when my body quit breathing on its own. Dr. Maguire was quite stoic and calm as he explained these events to me. He had a stillness and a quiet strength that silently conveyed that even he was surprised I had made it through the events and survived. I believe he was also deeply cognizant and in complete reverence of the awesome power that turned him around that day.

Over the years, I've often remembered the story he told me, as well as his words, "A power greater than me turned me around and told me that I had to at least try..." I have wondered, many times, how Dr. Maguire must have felt when, after the surgery, I quit breathing and had to be placed on the ventilator. Did he second guess his decision? I never really found the right opportunity to tell him that I couldn't thank

God enough for him and his decision. I wanted to somehow convey to him that I was intensely aware that he saved my life. I wanted to apologize if he agonized at all over his decision. I wanted to tell him that he was an angel to me and that I was beyond thankful for him. I realize he was just going about his usual day and doing his job, but I knew then and I know now that God led me to him. God closed every single door that didn't lead to him, because God knew he had the expertise to save my life. God also knew that Dr. Maguire was a man of faith. He was a man who would be moved by that awesome, silent power that created and controls the universe.

Again, those words, "A power greater than me turned me around and told me that I had to at least try…" have prompted me to continue trying many times in my life when I wanted to just give up. Those words cemented firmly in the depths of my soul the belief that God has a plan for me. We each have our own individual beliefs, but I believe, without a doubt, that God turned Dr. Maguire around that day. God had been a part of this process from the very beginning. I have to believe that if God kept me here, then I should do everything I can to fulfill my purpose on this planet.

For many years, however, I wasn't sure what that purpose was exactly. It's easy to get sidetracked in life and to start to believe that you're on the right path when you really are about as far off course as you could possibly get. During those moments, I have always felt God tapping me on my shoulder and reminding me that He saved me for a reason. And as my life has evolved, I realized that what my story is about is a suffering soul and the will to overcome the pain and agony encapsulating it.

I believe that I needed to walk down many paths, some of them easy, others far more difficult, some of them right and some of them drastically wrong, in order for me to be able to tell the story that needed to be told —the emotional journey that we experience when we don't fit into the mold that society considers attractive and acceptable.

At the root of our soul, hope is alive, begging to be released and begin its journey, attempting to ultimately deliver us to its intended destination of love, peace, and happiness. Along the way if we find the capability to listen in quiet solitude, we will hear the voice of God whispering, "I am here." He will prepare our way, open our needed doors, and sprinkle our path with angels to assist us.

There is so much more to being happy than arriving at your goal weight. The emotional journey involved in losing weight is just as important, if not more important, than the physical journey. I know so many people are in the same situation I was, thinking that if they lose the weight they will be happy again, plain and simple. Life doesn't work that way, though. Happy is a constantly evolving process in our lives. The canvas that is our story has been painted upon by every single person that has crossed our path in our lifetime. Regardless of how minimal their presence was, they have picked up their brush and added their touches to our picture. We decide how significant or insignificant their additions will be based on how we ultimately evolve in our own character.

"You must give everything to make your life as beautiful as the dreams that dance in your imagination."

—Roman Payne

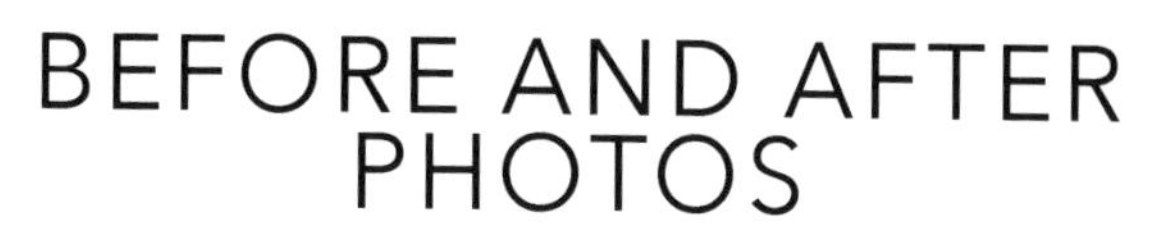

BEFORE AND AFTER PHOTOS

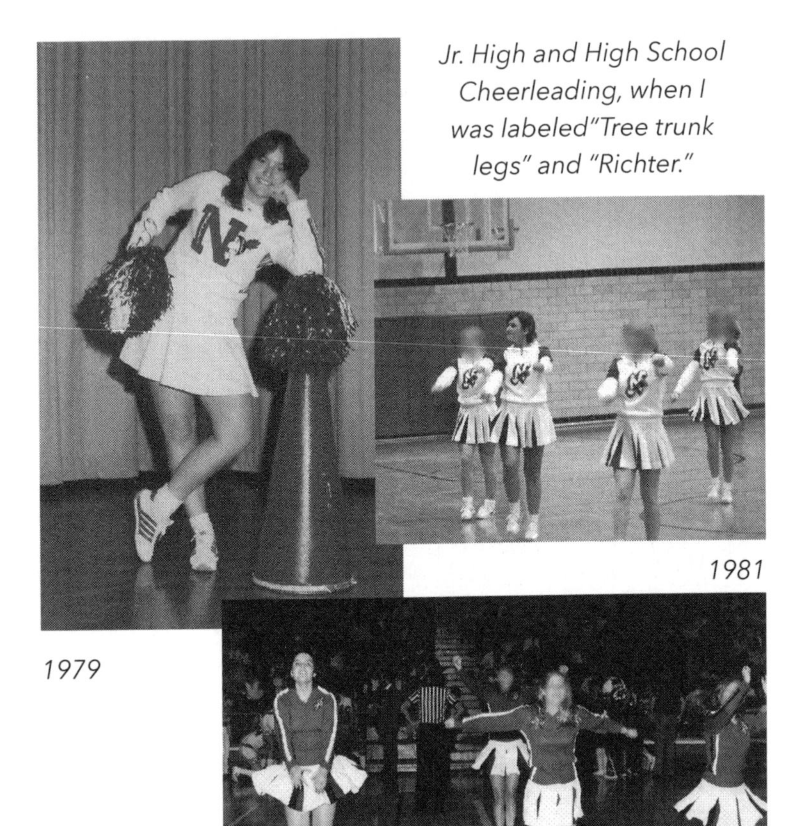

Jr. High and High School Cheerleading, when I was labeled"Tree trunk legs" and "Richter."

1981

1979

1982

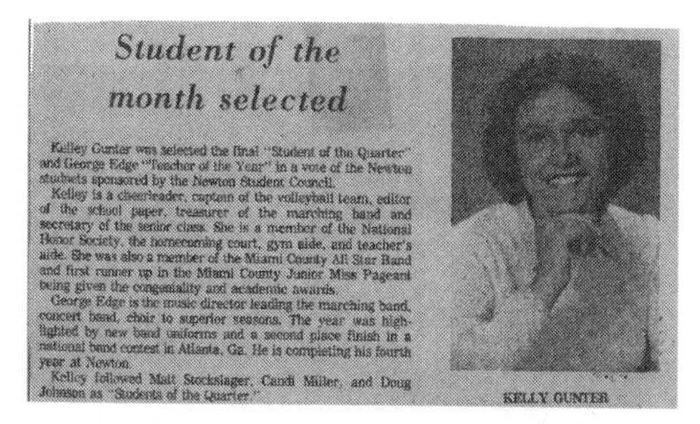

Student of the month selected

Kelley Gunter was selected the final "Student of the Quarter" and George Edge "Teacher of the Year" in a vote of the Newton students sponsored by the Newton Student Council.

Kelley is a cheerleader, captain of the volleyball team, editor of the school paper, treasurer of the marching band and secretary of the senior class. She is a member of the National Honor Society, the homecoming court, gym aide, and teacher's aide. She was also a member of the Miami County All Star Band and first runner up in the Miami County Junior Miss Pageant being given the congeniality and academic awards.

George Edge is the music director leading the marching band, concert band, choir to superior seasons. The year was highlighted by new band uniforms and a second place finish in a national band contest in Atlanta, Ga. He is completing his fourth year at Newton.

Kelley followed Matt Stockslager, Candi Miller, and Doug Johnson as "Students of the Quarter."

KELLY GUNTER

My constant drive for perfection was fueled by my poor self-image. It didn't matter what I accomplished, it was impossible to fill that void.

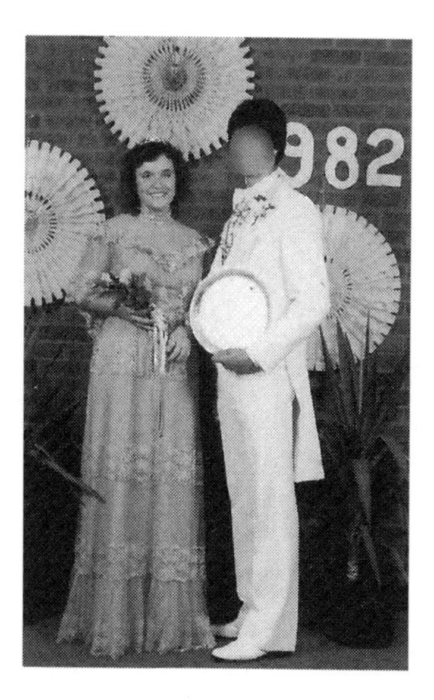

1982 Prom Princess

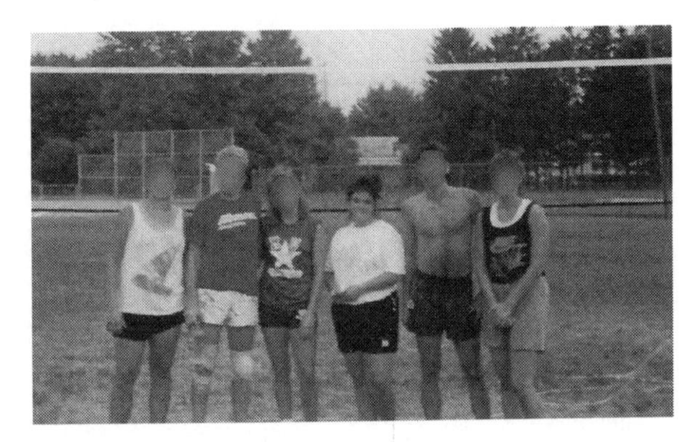

My College Years
1984-1988. I was gaining weight at a pretty rapid rate.

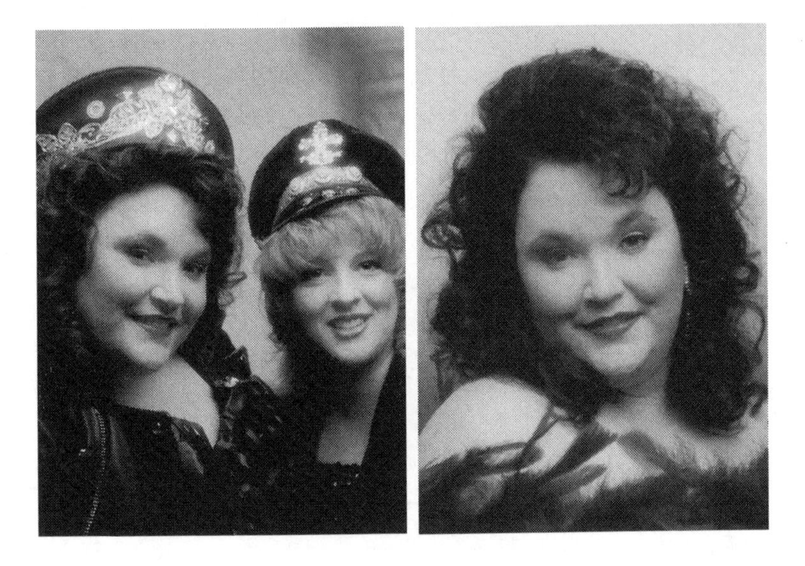

My best friend Lori and me, doing Glamour Shots

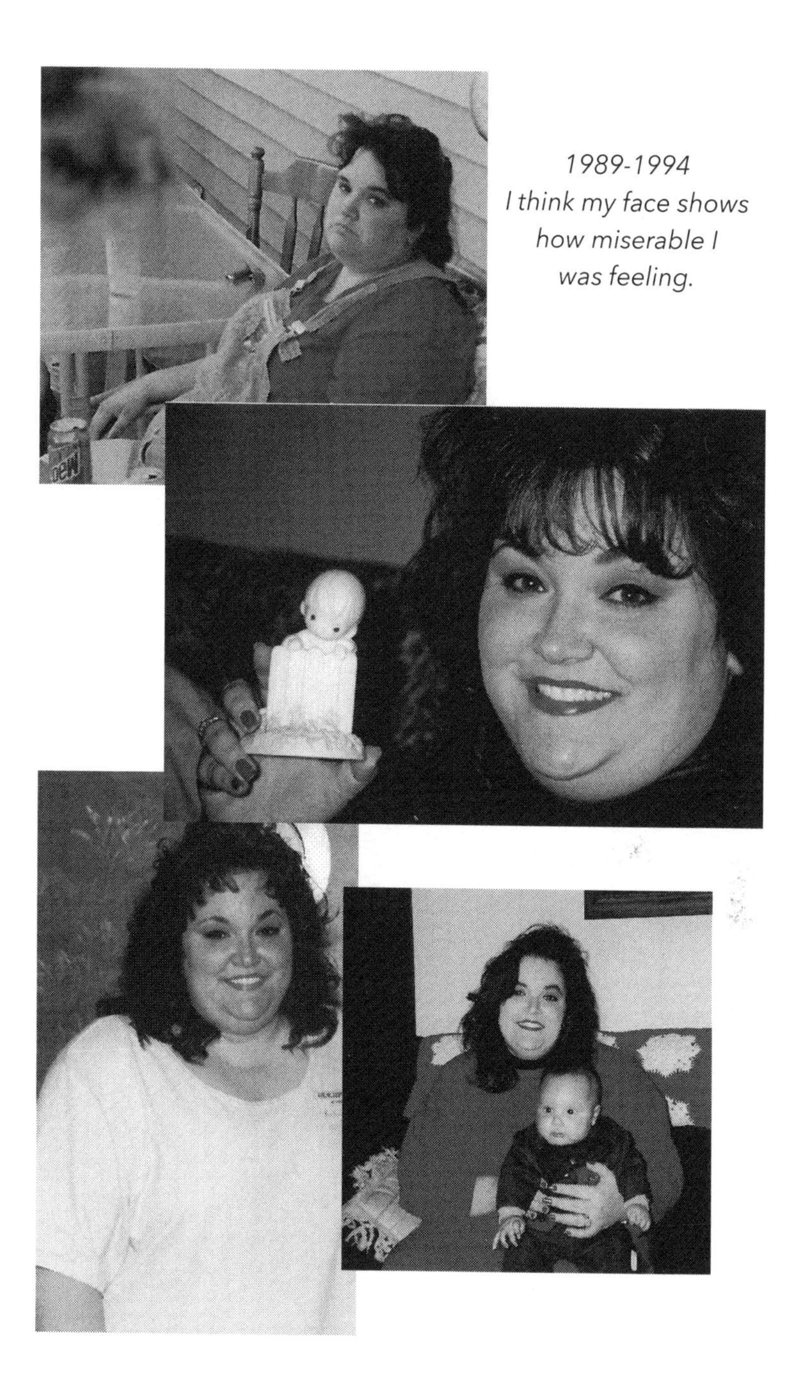

1989-1994
I think my face shows
how miserable I
was feeling.

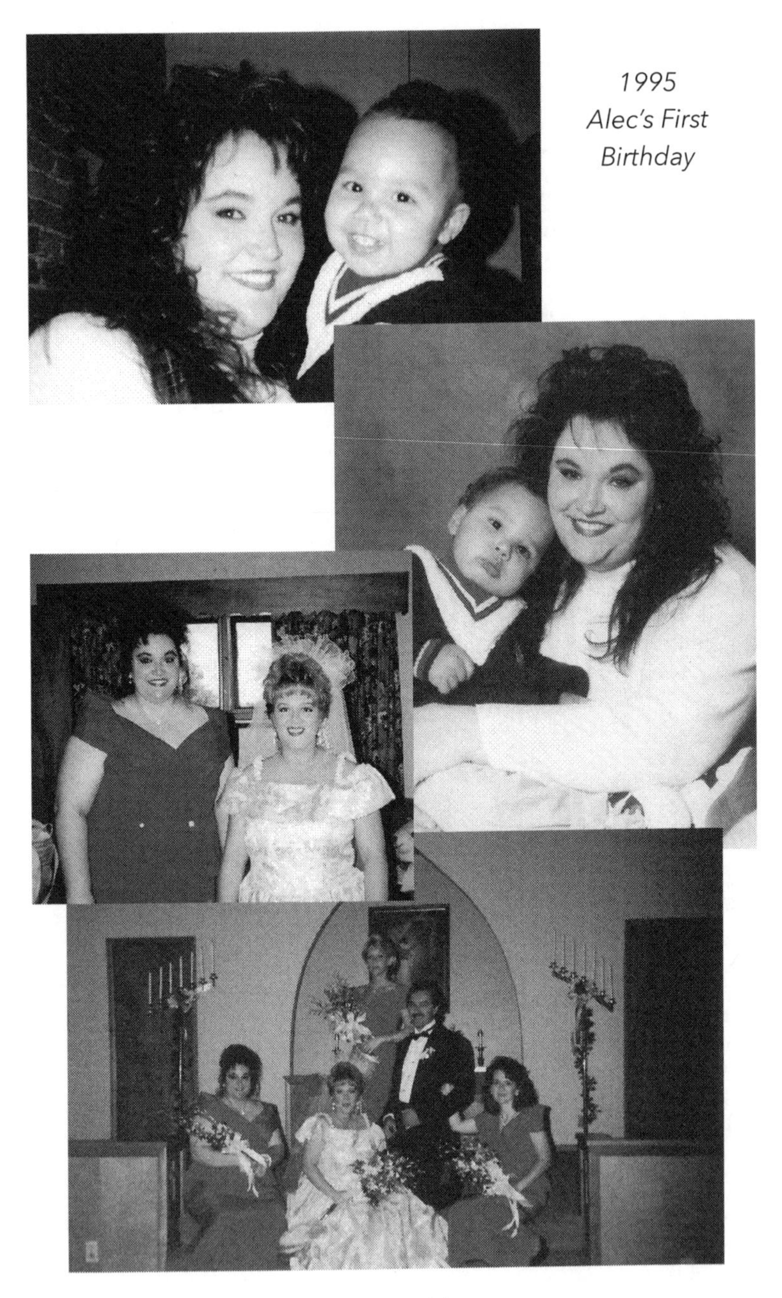

*1995
Alec's First
Birthday*

Lori's Wedding

1996-2002 | 391 lbs

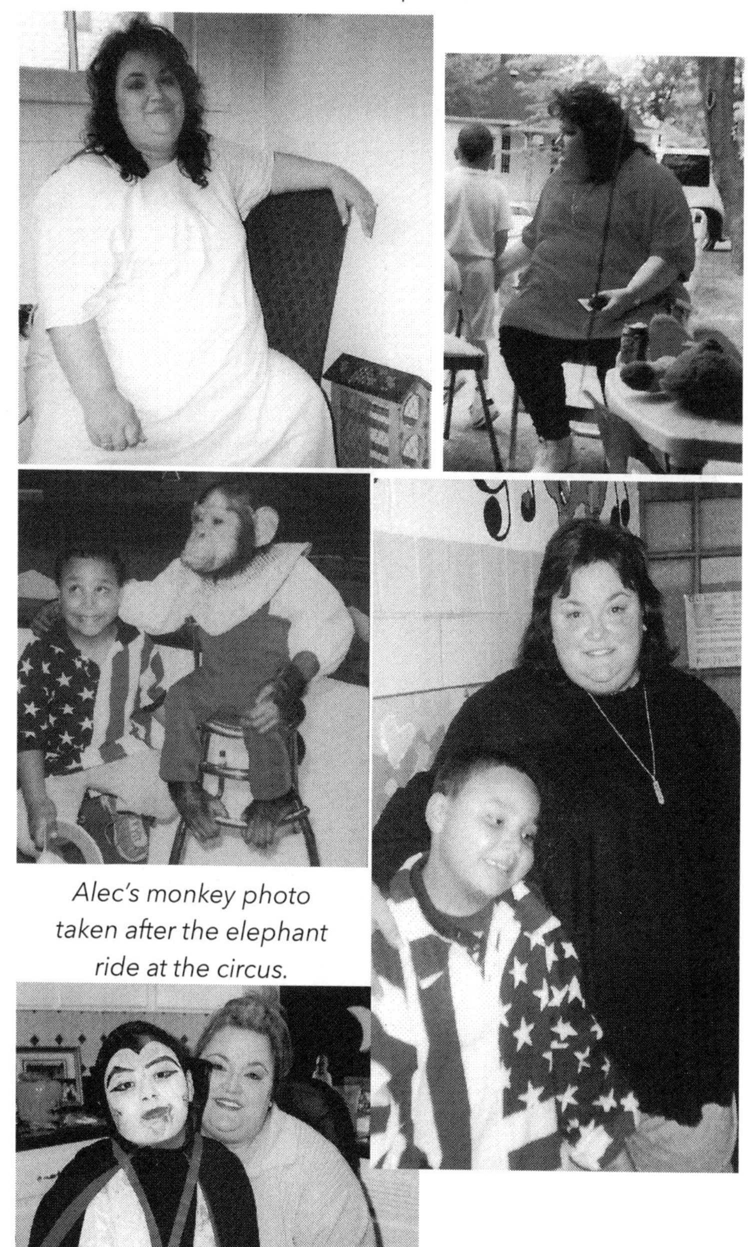

Alec's monkey photo taken after the elephant ride at the circus.

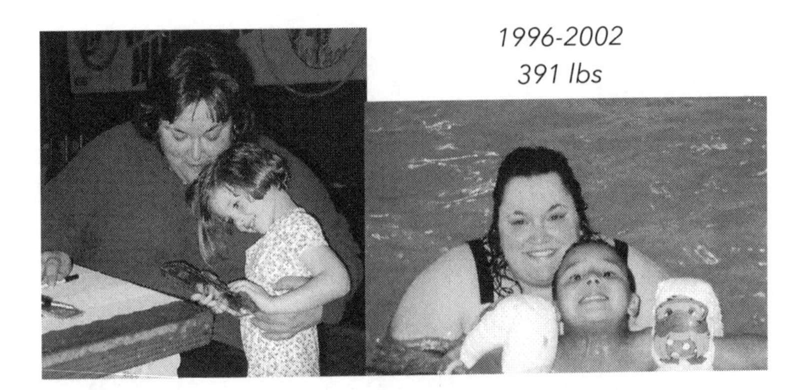

1996-2002
391 lbs

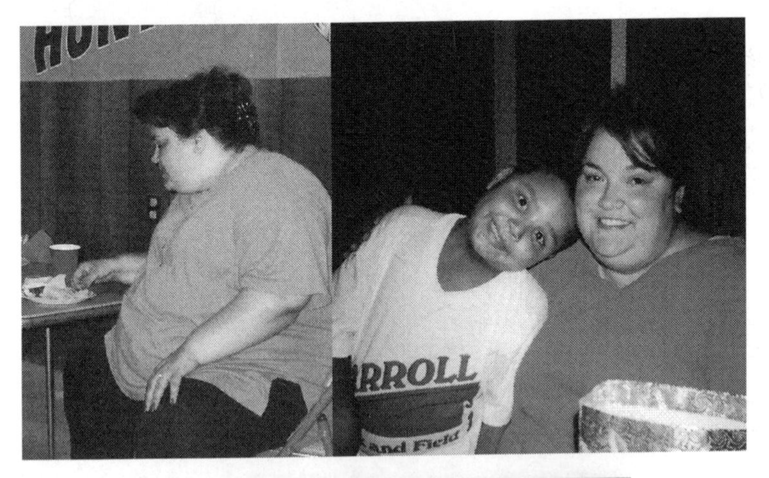

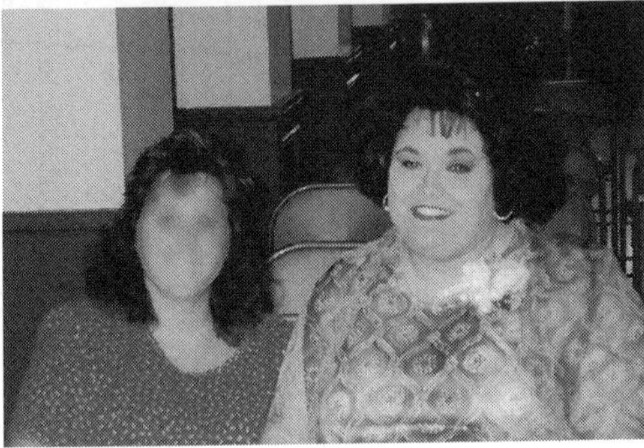

August 2002 - 391 lbs
Photos taken at Dr. Maguire's Office by his assistant Kim, a couple of days before my surgery on August 2, 2002.

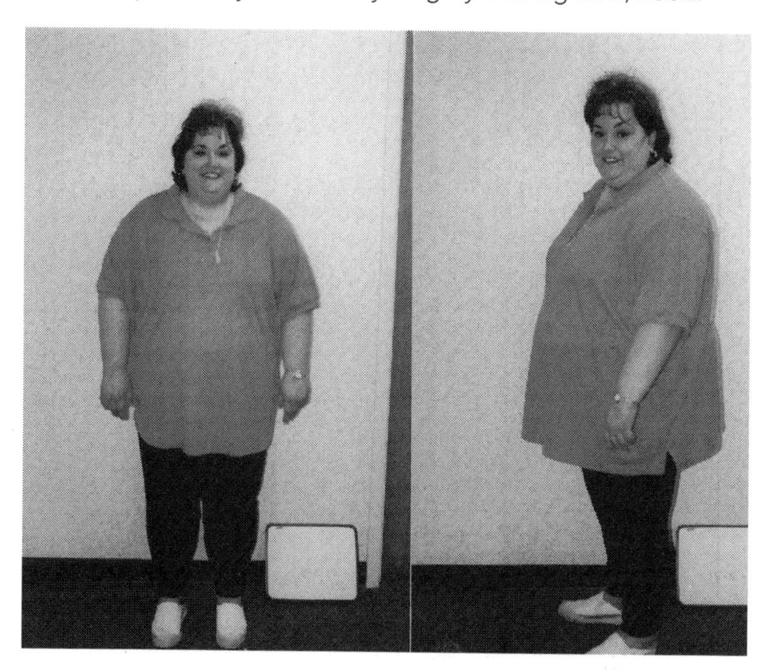

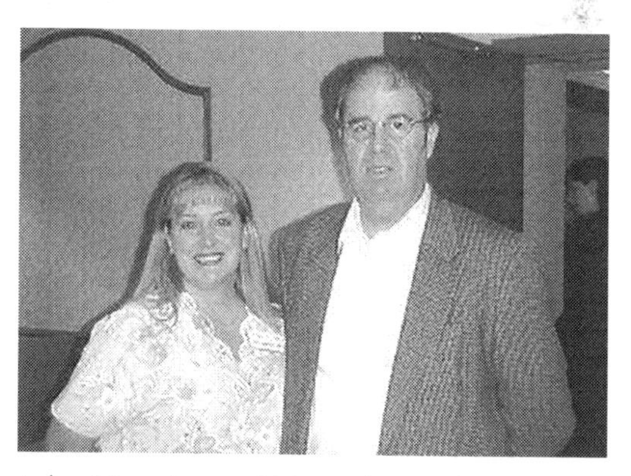

Dr. John Maguire and his assistant Kim, circa 2002.

Letters written by Dr. Gregg, Director of Critical Care at Kettering Hospital and Dr. Maguire that were part of my successful appeal to my insurance company.

SOUTH DAYTON SURGEONS INC

September 10, 2002

[illegible]

[illegible]

John P. Maguire M.D., F.A.C.S.

[illegible]

[illegible]

[illegible]

General, Vascular & Laparoscopic Surgery

RE: Kelley Gunter

To Whom It May Concern:

Dear Sirs:

Kelley Gunter underwent bariatric surgery for severe obesity. Kelley chose to undergo the duodenal switch operation rather than the Roux-en-Y gastric bypass. She thought it would be more likely to provide success for her long term based on her personality and lifestyle. She was aware that this was not covered by your insurance company and she did pay cash for this.

At the time of surgery she had hypertension and Floppy eye syndrome that were attributed to her obesity. At the time of surgery, however, we found she had a chronic abdominal compartment syndrome and developed respiratory failure postoperatively related to this. I feel the patient was much sicker than we even anticipated. She was on the verge of respiratory failure because of her severe obesity. This was diagnosed postoperatively and she probably also has sleep apnea. She has been on oxygen at home since surgery. Hopefully we will be able to get her off of this soon. She is feeling better after about 40 pounds of weight loss.

We would request that you provide coverage for her for the workup and treatment of her respiratory problem, which was present before surgery and not a result of the surgery. Thank you for consideration of this matter.

Sincerely,

John P. Maguire, M.D.

JPM/ts

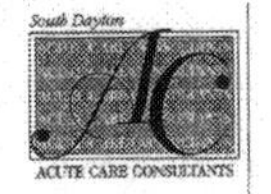

South Dayton AC ACUTE CARE CONSULTANTS

CRITICAL CARE MEDICINE

Robert Barker, M.D.

Jorge Crespo, M.D.

Richard Gregg, M.D.

Shachi Rattan, M.D.

INFECTIOUS DISEASES

Jorge Crespo, M.D.

James Galbraith, M.D.

Jeffrey Weinstein, M.D.

Howard Wunderlich, M.D.

Talal Zreik, M.D.

INTERNAL MEDICINE

Chacko Alappatt, M.D.

Stephen Lucht, M.D.

Mark Marinella, M.D.

Gary J. Palmer, M.D.

Indu Rao, M.D.

Wendy Schmitz, M.D.

Melody Singer, M.D.

33 West Rahn Road

Suite #102

Dayton, Ohio 45429

PH: (937) 433-8990

Fax: (937) 433-8691

www.adacc.com

September 23, 2002

Medical Director
Anthem / Community Choice
P O Box 37180
Louisville, KY 40233 7180

RE: Kelley Gunter #61495
DOB 03/14/65

Dear Medical Director:

I understand that Anthem is considering denial of Kelley Gunter's hospital stay from August 5 to August 11, 2002. As a medical director, I share your concern regarding unwarranted hospital stays and excess costs. However, I would certainly encourage review of this instance.

Ms. Gunter is a 37-year-old woman with morbid obesity. She underwent biliopancreatic diversion with duodenal switch, appendectomy, cholecystectomy and J-tube placement by Dr. Maguire. Her situation was complicated by difficulty breathing in the recovery room. She was given Decadron and epinephrine without much improvement and ultimately required reintubation. We were asked to participate in her care regarding her mechanical ventilation and ICU stay.

She did have a history of hypertension, but no known particular cardiac problem. However, her preoperative pO2 was 76 and pulmonary function testing had shown mixed obstructive and restrictive pulmonary disease. She apparently had frequent wheezing and was dyspneic walking less than 100 yards.

She was admitted to the ICU and over time, she was weaned, extubated and ultimately dismissed. Clearly in this setting, her inpatient stay was warranted.

We appreciate your review of this claim.

Sincerely,

Richard W. Gregg, MD, FACP, FCCP, FCCM

rg/cm

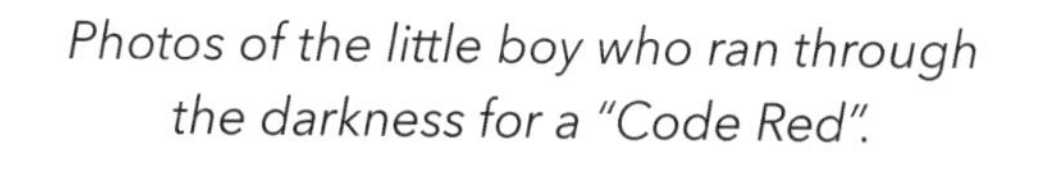

Photos of the little boy who ran through the darkness for a "Code Red".

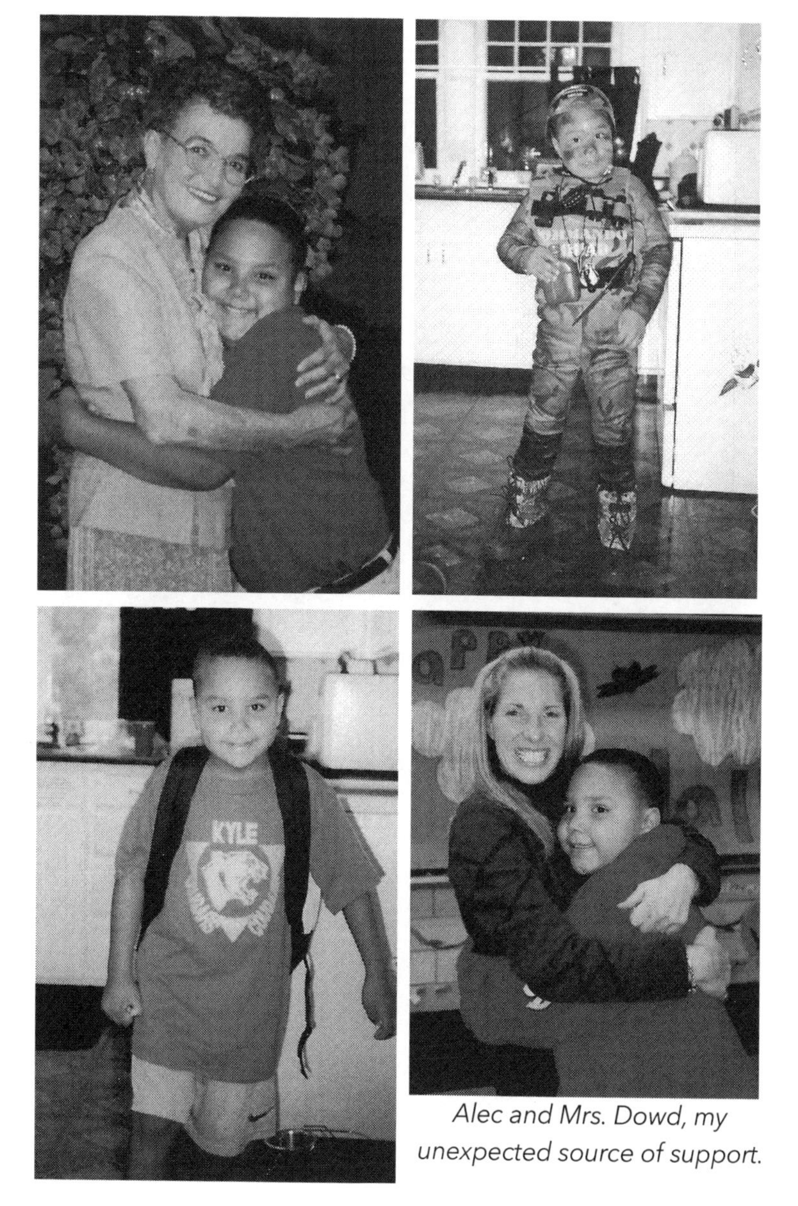

Alec and Mrs. Dowd, my unexpected source of support.

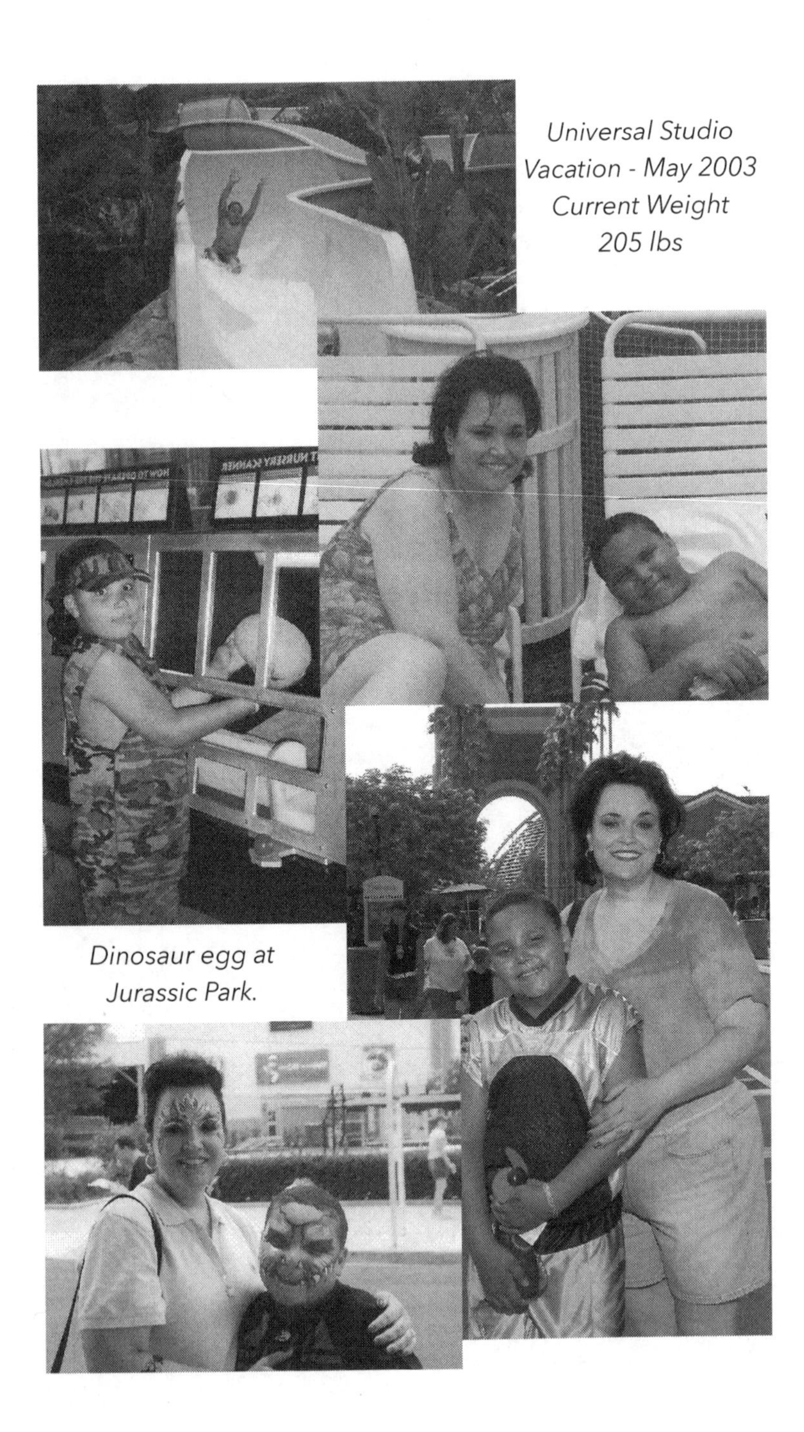

Universal Studio
Vacation - May 2003
Current Weight
205 lbs

Dinosaur egg at
Jurassic Park.

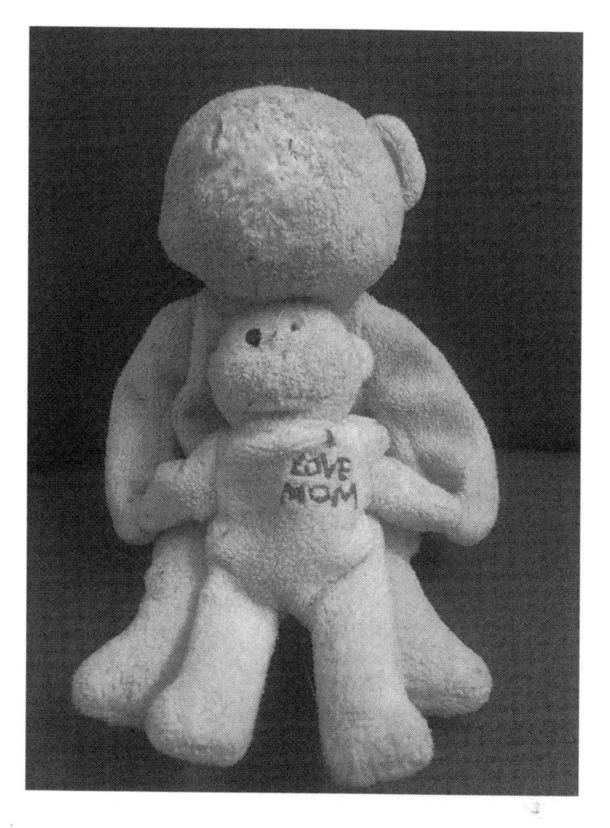

"my 'loved out' bears....beautiful and perfect"

First plastic surgery - excess skin removal - November 2003 Body Lift/thigh lift by Dr. Jose Berger

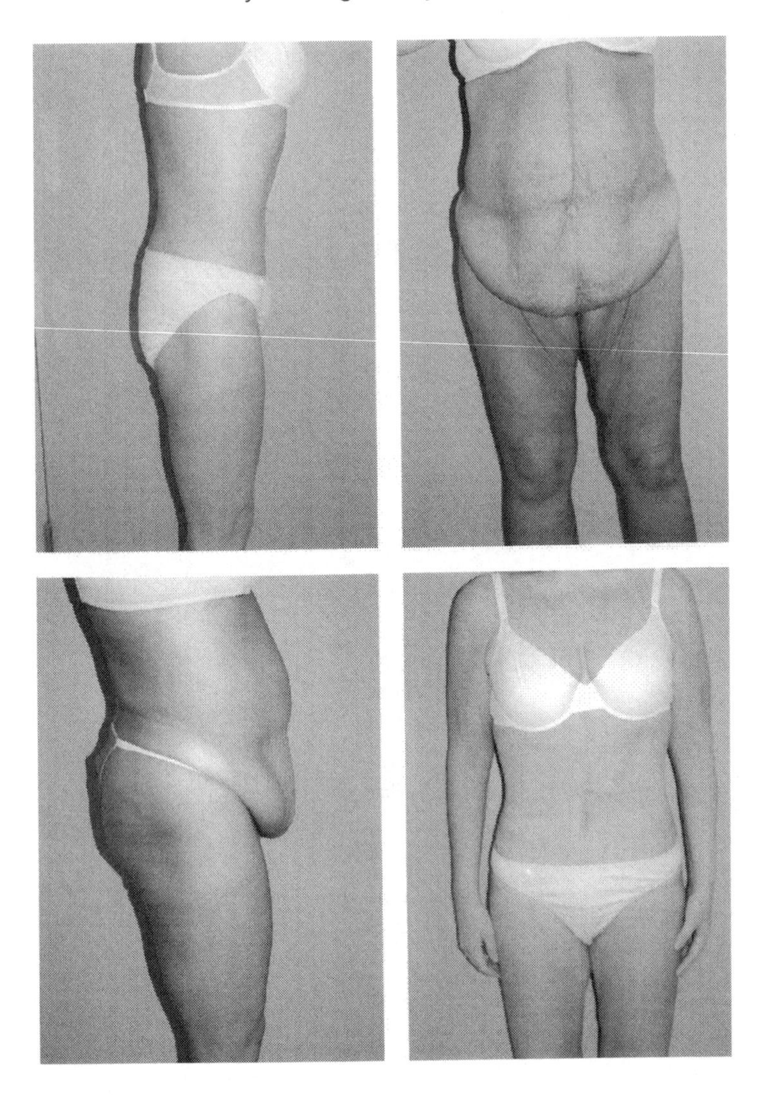

Dear mommy I love
you alot and I
hope you get well
soon.

love,
Alec Günter Huffman.
a k a the [illegible]

A note from Alec that I found on my pillow after I returned home from plastic surgery.

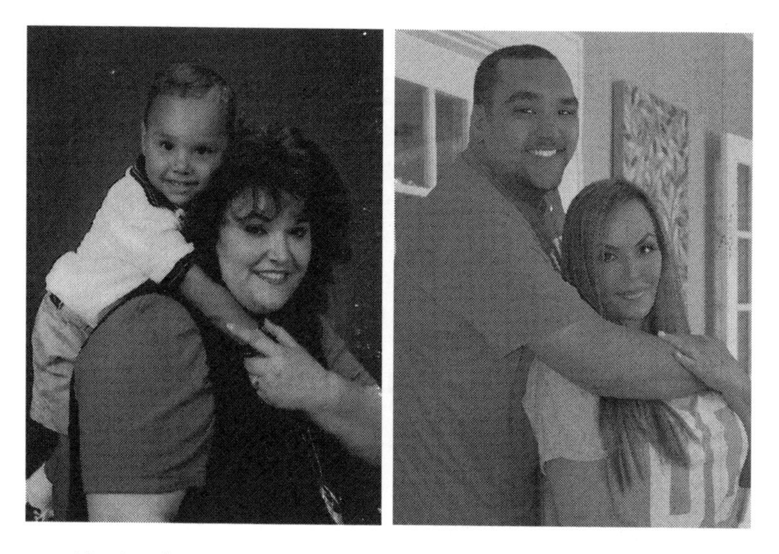

Alec and me, October 1997. Alec and me, August 2017

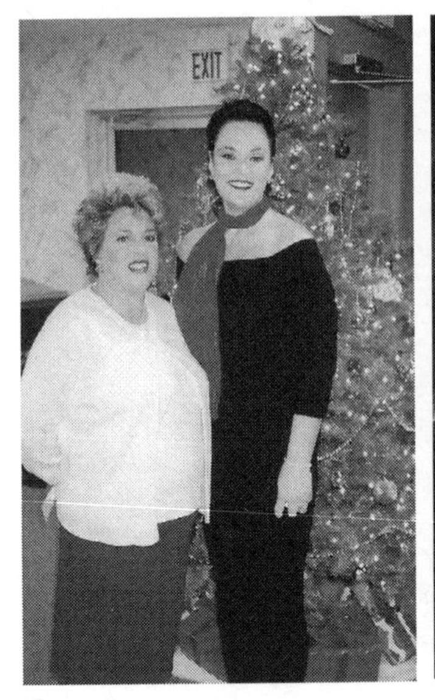

December 2004
Lori and me at Alec's
Piano Recital.

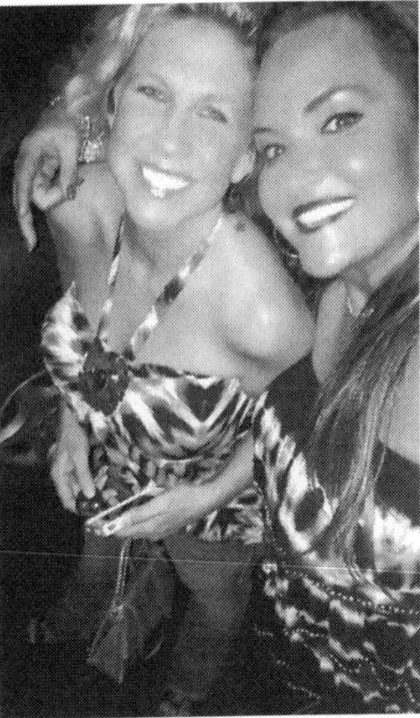

August 2013
Amy and me enjoying
a girl's night out.

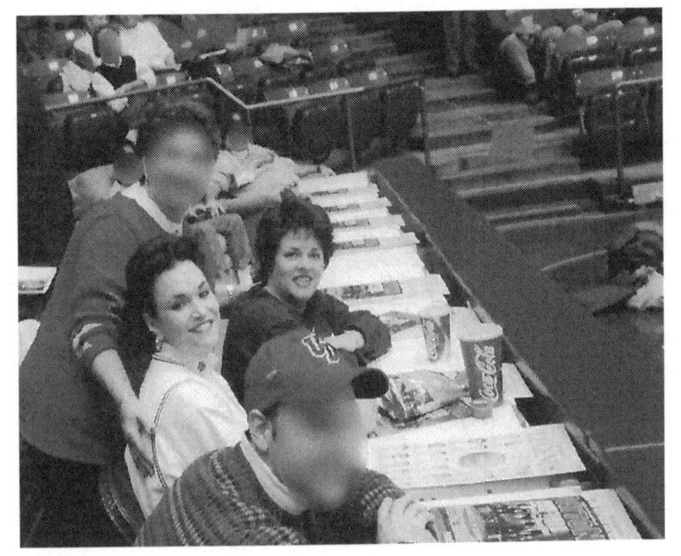

Winter 2005 -
Lori and me at a University of Dayton Basketball Game.

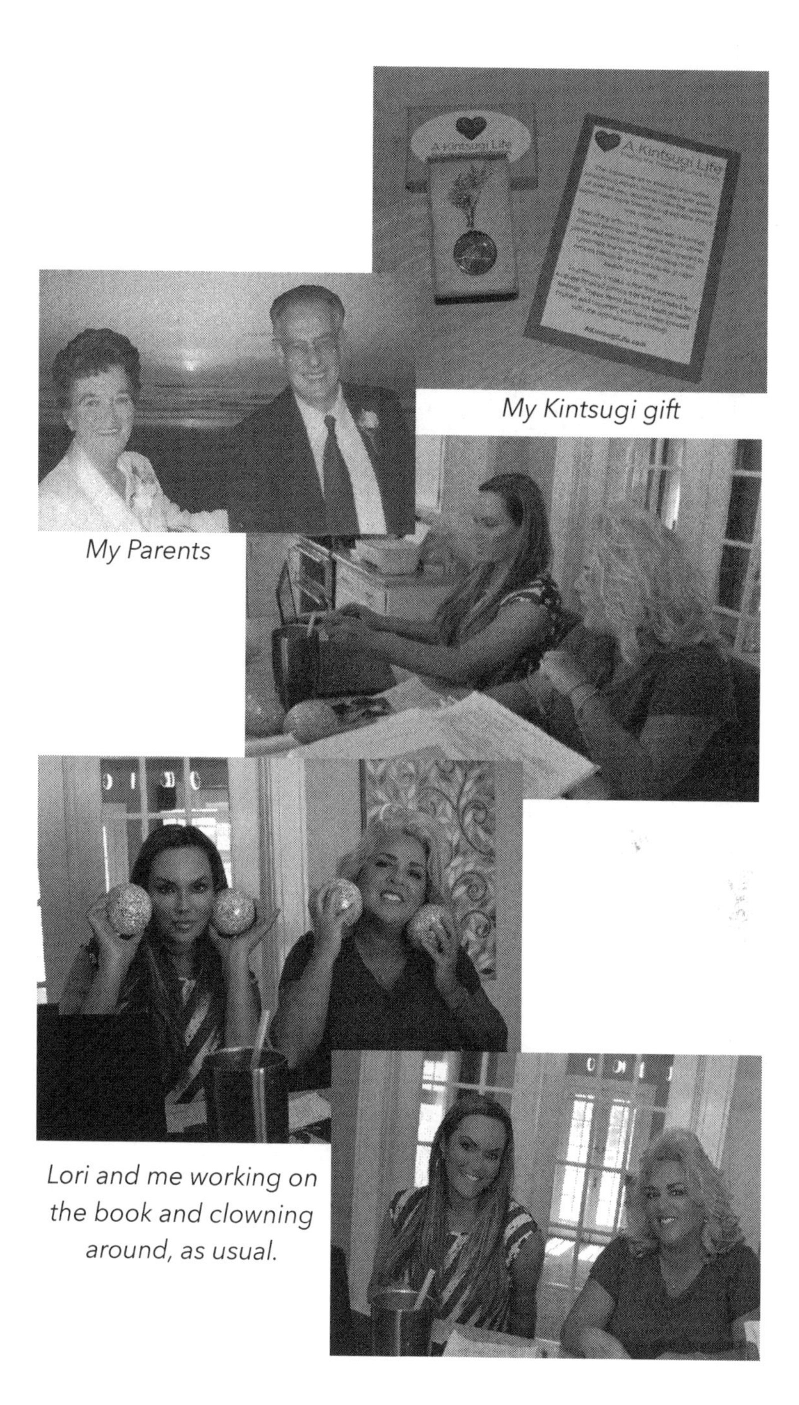

My Kintsugi gift

My Parents

Lori and me working on the book and clowning around, as usual.

2016 -2017

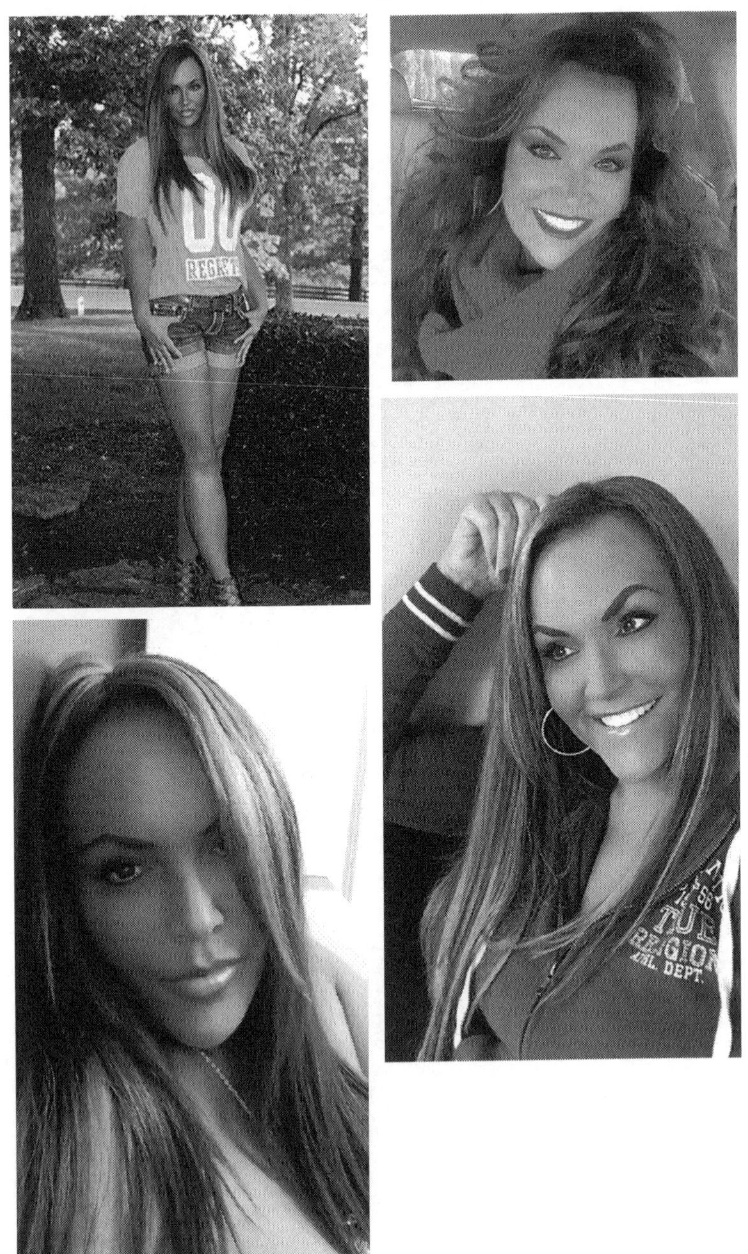

2016 -2017

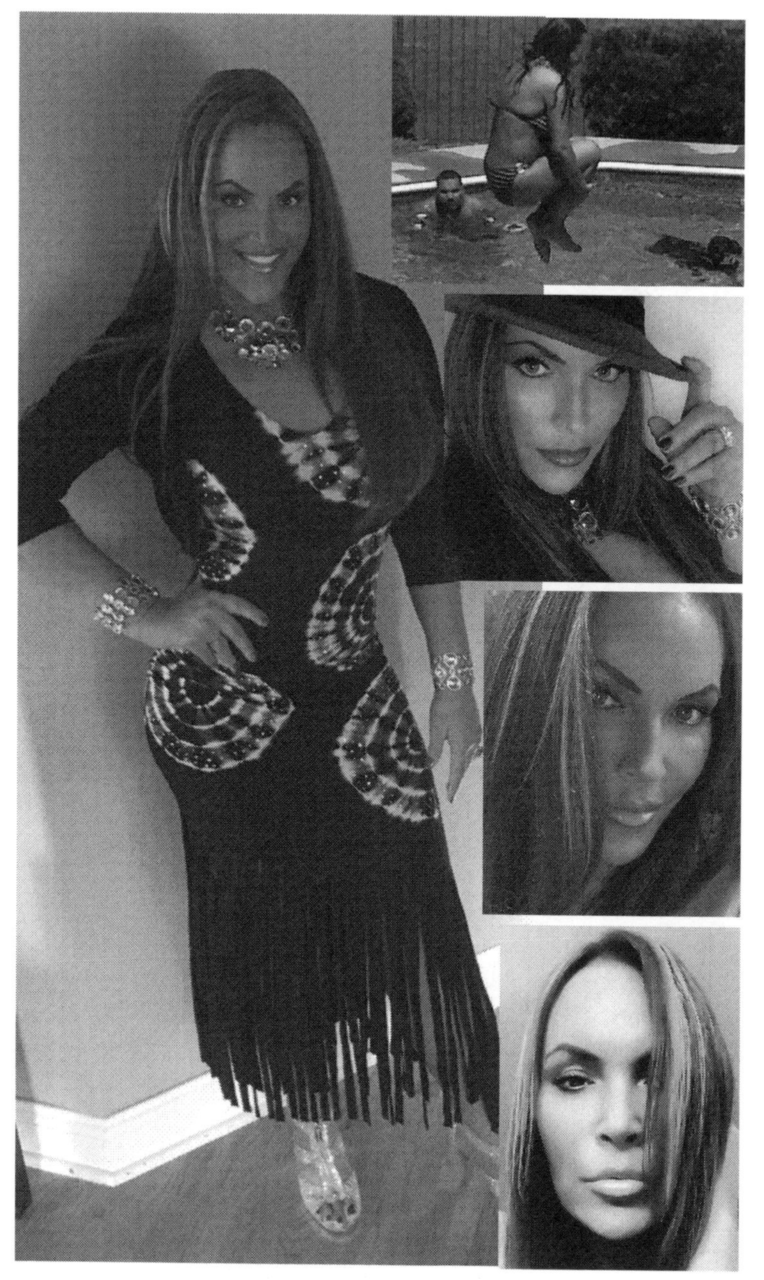

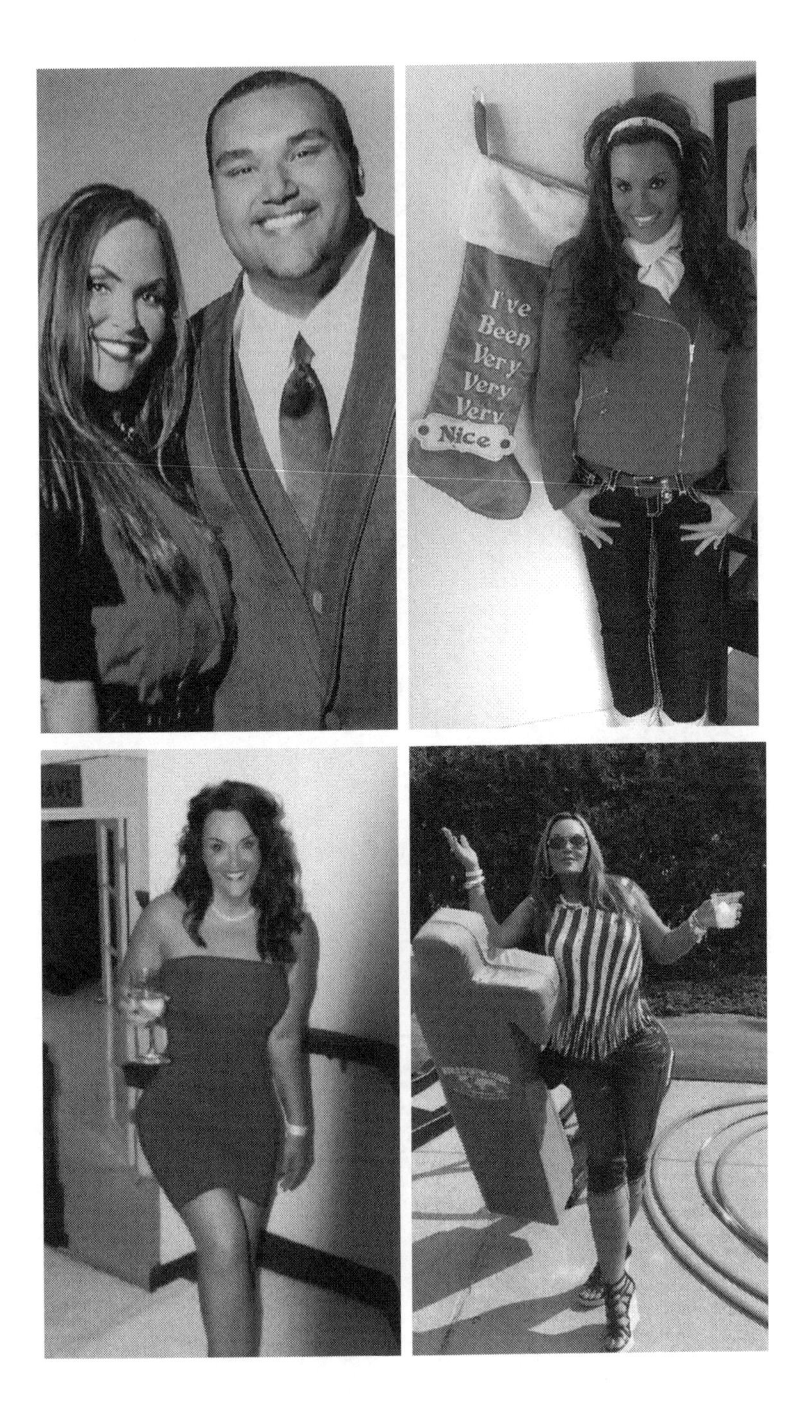
I've
Been
Very
Very
Very
Nice

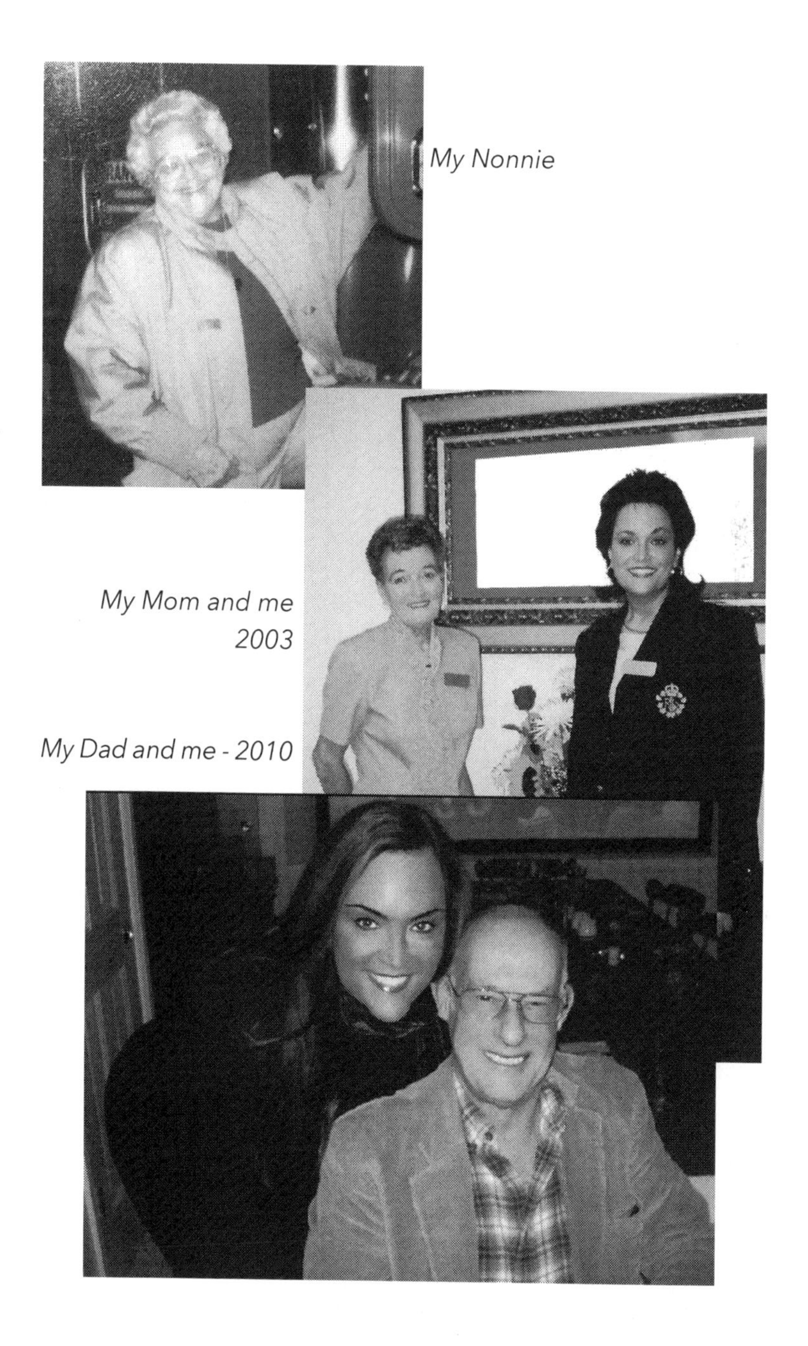

My Nonnie

My Mom and me
2003

My Dad and me - 2010

PART II

"Not until we are lost do we begin to understand ourselves."

—Henry David Thoreau

CHAPTER 7

"We delight in the beauty of the butterfly, but rarely admit the changes it has gone through to achieve that beauty.

—Maya Angelou

I was home. I was in pain and misery. Even though I expected to be uncomfortable after the surgery, I wasn't prepared for what I was experiencing. In spite of the fact that the morphine drip I had at the hospital made me a lunatic, I was wishing I had some of that at home. Acting nutty seemed like a better option than being in agony. I've never been a tough girl when it came to pain, and this was no exception. My poor family had their hands full.

My incision was huge and painful, and I still had tubes everywhere. In spite of being on oxygen, I still felt as though I could barely breathe. Moving the slightest amount hurt. When I did summon up the courage to move, it felt as though

I was going to burst wide open. I had stitches, staples, and huge plastic clips with wires keeping my incision together. I still had a PICC line in my neck, just in case I needed fluids or nutrition long-term. Dr. Maguire had told us in the surgery orientation that we would be uncomfortable when we came home. The word uncomfortable doesn't even begin to describe how I felt.

It was incredibly hard for me to sit up in my bed. I couldn't get myself into a sitting position without assistance. Thankfully I had a canopy bed, and my dad was very handy. He created a device that hung over the top of the canopy, similar to the ones on hospital beds. I could reach up and grab it to help pull myself up into a seated position. That little contraption helped me so much. It was like a miracle. It has since occurred to me that on a day-to-day basis we tend to take thousands of little things for granted. Who knew sitting up in bed could become so difficult? It's uncanny that as humans, many times it's only when we lose the ability to do something or have something, that we place significance on it.

When I came into my room that first night, I found a little gift on my pillow from my son. It was a stuffed mommy teddy bear, holding a little baby bear on her lap. On the little teddy bear's stomach was, "I love Mom." It was the perfect size to hold in my hands. Alec had picked it out for me at the store and wanted me to have it when I came home. I slept with that bear and hung onto it every night. It was my little source of comfort and love. I would hold it close to me and think of my son and the reason why I was fighting so hard to survive and get healthy. Over the last 15 years those bears have absorbed so many tears.

Those little teddy bears were my secret portal for strength and courage and reminded me of all the reasons I had the surgery, all the things and people I was fighting for. Those bears reminded me of what was truly important, love. Those bears traveled with me everywhere. When I had to leave town without my son, I took those bears with me and slept with them every single night. My friends and colleagues would laugh at me and tease me about those bears, but I didn't care one bit. If I was going somewhere, those bears were going as well. Those bears have traveled to many, many places. I still have them. They have the look of having been deeply loved. At one point their faces were chewed off by an overzealous Rottweiler puppy, but I didn't discard them, I found people to help me patch them back together. That's what love does. Many people would look at them and say that they were old, dirty, and that they had outlived their time. But I look at them and see the true portrait of strength, survival, and genuine love.

Isn't that the true portrait of love? When I see a toy or a stuffed animal that looks like that, my first thought is, "Wow!!!! That has been LOVED !!!" I hope that when I reach the Pearly Gates and St. Peter gets a look at me, I look as though I have been deeply loved. I hope I show so much wear and tear that it is obvious I was someone's source of comfort and support. I want to be physical proof of how many people wanted to have me in their presence for laughter and light.

Just like those battered teddy bears, I hope my hands are worn and show the evidence of how many people held onto them. I hope I have stains on me indicative of all the times spent enjoying love and laughter during all the wonderful meals I've shared with the people I loved. I pray my ears are almost nonexistent because I used them so much listening to others, and my eyes are tired from trying to see another's pain. And I pray that my heart is literally falling into pieces because I used it so much and gave love to so many people. Yes, I hope I wear my heart out just like those two little bears that were forever attached together in the same way a mother and her son are connected. In fact, I don't call that worn out, I call that "loved out" and in my book, that's an incredibly beautiful thing.

With my bears in my hand, I struggled with how much I hurt and the fact that I couldn't eat anything without vomiting. And as you can imagine, vomiting only made the pain worse. My surgery had greatly reduced the size of my stomach. Because of that, I would get full so quickly, I could only eat a few bites at a time. When I first came home, I felt like I was starving. I'm not sure if that was an emotional or a physical hunger, but one of the first things I asked for was some peanut butter toast. Jeff brought me two pieces and I ate one bite, pushed the plate away and said I was full. His response was, "Yeah, right." I was thankful my mom was still sitting there and she explained to him that my stomach was literally that small for now, and I couldn't eat very much at one time.

The fact that I couldn't eat like I used to presented a major difficulty for me. I had been using food as a comfort for the last several years. When I was sad, angry, depressed, or even happy, I would eat. The emotion really didn't matter, food and eating was my way of dealing with it. We've all seen in the movies the heart-broken girl who has just been dumped, tears streaming down her face, spoon in hand, diving into a gallon of ice cream. It's a way of self-medicating, it's pain reliever straight from the freezer. But I couldn't do that anymore. My stomach wouldn't allow me. It was way too small for that. Suddenly all of those questions the doctor asked me during the psychological evaluation were making sense. How was I going to deal with my emotions when I couldn't use food?

At this point, however, I couldn't even think about food, because I was in too much pain and vomiting so much that I didn't care. I had a potty chair beside the bed because it was incredibly difficult for me to walk all the way to the bathroom. I didn't like the potty chair. I didn't like sitting on that thing in the middle of my bedroom. I felt so exposed. My miniature schnauzer Sparky would look at me, and I imagined by his expression that he was saying, "*What* are you doing?" To avoid the embarrassment and unease on most occasions I insisted on walking all the way to the bathroom. This was not an easy task and even more difficult for those taking care of me due to my various equipment. One thing the potty chair was good for was providing a convenient place for me to vomit. Since I was vomiting all day long, it came in quite handy.

Something I believe people need to understand is that having weight loss surgery is not the easy way out that some misguidedly claim it to be. There is nothing easy about surgical weight loss. Regardless of how one chooses to lose weight, it is not an easy venture. I've seen a few national magazines with covers of before and after weight loss pictures where the headlines read, "No weight loss surgery, no tricks or gimmicks… no easy way out…" Again, there is nothing easy about weight loss surgery. Each of us search to find a way that works for us. I applaud anyone who has the courage to make their journey work for them. I can celebrate anyone's victory without adding a qualifier that makes them feel like they cheated or took a shortcut. Just because someone achieved their goal in a different way than I did doesn't make their victory any less satisfying and worthy of praise.

There were countless times in the first month that I regretted having the surgery. I was so miserable, and I would just sit and question why I ever did this. I would tell myself I must have really been a fool to have had this surgery. I couldn't imagine living the rest of my life this way. I would think to myself that I should have just stayed fat and that I could have lost the weight if I tried harder. I must have said to my friends and my family a hundred times, "I shouldn't have had this surgery." Of course, there were the friends who would say that they knew this would happen and they tried to tell me and that I should have listened to them and that this was a bad idea. But then there were the soldiers in my life, the inner circle if you will, who told me that it was going to get better and that this was just a difficult beginning. They reminded me that nothing great is created suddenly, and that I really wouldn't know if it was a success for about a year. They encouraged me and they believed in me. They didn't let me stay doubtful for long.

Here's my advice for anyone considering surgery or any major life decision. If you have negative people on your roster, cut them from your team now. No one who is in your corner is going to feed your mind with negativity. Thoughts become reality, and you need to fill your team with positive people who believe in you. In those dark, difficult moments when you doubt yourself or your decision, it is essential you have people who truly want the best for you. You don't need people who have hidden agendas, secret jealousy, or who have their own issues that they are trying to take out on you. I learned the hard way that some people only say that they're trying to help you. Weed those people out. You deserve better.

After about a month, when I felt up to it, I did as Dr.

Gregg had instructed me and I obtained letters from him, Dr. Maguire, and my family physician, Dr. Goodenough, regarding my unknown, severe medical condition prior to surgery. I sent the letters in with my formal appeal to my insurance company, asking them to reimburse Kettering Hospital for all of the expenses they incurred providing my extraordinary, life-saving care. My first appeal was denied rather quickly. I filed a second appeal, and it, too, was denied expeditiously. It certainly appeared as though my insurance simply wasn't going to acquiesce in regards to their refusal to pay for my surgery, even though it clearly had saved my life. They would only consider three appeals and I'd already lost my first two. I honestly didn't think it was worth trying again, but I went ahead and completed the paperwork and submitted it as a third and final appeal. All I could do was wait for their response.

In the meantime, for the first several months following my surgery, I felt as though I had swallowed a little man who had a trampoline and he was residing in my stomach. Everything I ate, that little man bounced right back up and out of my stomach. It didn't matter what it was, it was most likely coming back up. I vomited so much, none of my friends or family even noticed anymore. One time we had a new friend over for dinner, and in the middle of the meal, I got up quickly from the table and went to the bathroom to get sick. I heard the friend asking what was wrong and my son said without any concern at all, "Oh, nothing, she's just getting sick. She does that all the time."

My BFF Lori was so accustomed to my being sick that it didn't faze her at all anymore. We were at another of our UD Basketball games. We always liked to be in our seats prior to the team coming out. The team came out onto the floor to the song, "Let's Get Ready to Rumble," and all of the fans would stand up and clap. It was an exciting part of the event. We had gotten something to eat prior to the game and I was in the bathroom, of course, getting sick. Lori was waiting for me outside by the mirrors, and in a rather rushed tone she said, "Are you done throwing up yet? Hurry up. We're going to miss, "Let's Get Ready to Rumble." I hurried myself as best I could, and when I opened the stall of the bathroom I saw all these ladies looking at Lori like she was a crazy person. As we walked down the steps to our seats we laughed and laughed about how they probably thought she was a terrible friend for saying those things to me. But she was just used to it. Everyone in my life was used to it. It was a part of my life at that point. It didn't even bother me anymore. If it went down, it was coming back up; or at least some of it was.

Remember that angel Kim, Dr. Maguire's nurse? Bless her heart, again. On one particularly trying day, I had tried to eat some garden-fresh tomatoes, because I loved them so much. Well, let me tell you, that the little man with the trampoline did not like the tomatoes one bit, and he bounced them up with a vengeance. I was having a bad day anyway, and that sent me over the edge. I grabbed my tiara and the Homecoming Queen of Crazy Town came back with a vengeance.

I grabbed my loving cup, my sash, and again, my reign was in full swing. I was in emotional turmoil and I just knew no one understood how I felt. I didn't want to hear one more rational explanation. I didn't want to hear another person tell me to calm down and that this wasn't going to be easy. I was tired of throwing up, tired of hurting, and tired of being on pain meds that made me crazy. I was tired of it all. For the love of everything holy, all I wanted was to eat a damn garden-fresh tomato and not have it propelled out of my stomach with the force of a tidal wave. Was that too much to ask?

I picked up the phone and I called Dr. Maguire's office. As you can imagine, I had the number memorized. I stopped sobbing long enough to ask for Kim and give my name. I'm certain the lady who answered the phone could tell I was crying, but she probably didn't realize I was hysterical. I was a tomato-eating fool and I was at war with this man in my stomach. He was clearly winning the battle, and this was the straw that broke the camel's back. I don't know what I thought I was going to accomplish, but the little man had to go.

Kim picked up the phone and as soon as I heard her voice, I began sobbing. In her calm manner she said, "Kelley, take a deep breath. What happened?" She just listened as I told her the horrific details of my most recent loss with the little obstinate vagrant who had begun residing in my abdomen. I went on and on about the fresh tomatoes and how much I loved them, and how I was tired of throwing up, and that I should have never had this surgery. Blah, blah, blah. Kim continued to listen quietly. Once I had stopped long enough to breathe and continue quietly crying she said, "Listen to me, a year from now you're going to be a size 8 and this will all be worth it." I let those words sink in for a few seconds. I took a deep breath and I asked, "But will I be eating fresh tomatoes?" She laughed a very deep, genuine laugh and she said, "Yes, Kelley, you will be eating fresh tomatoes."

Imagine if in the middle of your busy work day, you had to take a phone call from a hysterical nutbar like me. Even worse, imagine if that nutbar was calling you not just to cry, but to sob hysterically about not being able to eat one of her favorite foods. But guess which line in life Kim stands in? She stands in the line of people who get it. Kim understood that I wasn't really crying about the tomatoes. I was crying because all of the severe changes I was experiencing were difficult for me, and the one avenue I had always walked to handle stress, was now closed to me. Kim could have always put my call into voicemail or she could have told the receptionist to tell me that she would call me back, but she didn't. She always took the time to attempt to lessen my pain and to lower my stress. People who deal with others in that fashion are actually quite rare. I was never oblivious to the kindness she radiated.

Vomiting wasn't the only physical issue I had to deal with. As my body was adjusting to the surgery and all the internal changes involved, I also had severe diarrhea. In fact, I usually had both. On more than one occasion I would vomit and have diarrhea at the same time. On those occasions, I was a mess. I felt terrible, and even though I couldn't control it, it was still embarrassing. I would just begin crying uncontrollably. Jeff was such a wonderful support to me at this time. He had volunteered to stay and take care of me during the week, (with my mom's help, of course), and he went home on the weekends. This also allowed him to spend a lot of extended time with our son as well.

My parents, next door, took care of me while he was gone. Although the romantic relationship between Jeff and I had ended five years prior, he was still willing to help me and take care of me under the worst of situations. Even though our relationship couldn't work, that core of love was still present, and we would do anything to help each other. Love may not always work out in the way we initially hoped it would, but that doesn't mean it still can't be the most powerful force on the universe.

This man cleaned up my diarrhea and my vomit, bathed me, took care of me, and all the while, took care of our son as well. He dealt with my emotional meltdowns, mood swings, and constant crying because I was in pain. This weak-stomached man who had passed out during my delivery room C-section came through for me when I needed it most.

I'll never forget one particular day. I had been very sick, and Jeff had just bathed me, cleaned up the potty chair, changed the sheets on the bed, and had gotten me back into the bed for a nap. Alec came casually walking into my room and said, "Hi Mommy. Daddy is throwing up over the side of the front porch again." We laugh about that to this day. He never wanted me to know that he was getting sick every single time he was cleaning up my messes, and there were several messes a day. It takes an incredibly special person to care for someone on that level.

Allow me to say again, that there is nothing easy about weight loss surgery. I realize that I was not a simple weight loss patient. I had many serious health issues and had to fight just to survive. I'm sure that some people who had the same surgery I had encounter fewer problems and have an easier initial recovery than I did. I know since I had my surgery 15 years ago, several different versions of weight loss surgery have been developed, and many have far fewer side effects than mine did. I don't know about their success rates, but I can say that I am absolutely happy that I had the specific surgery I had. The only thing I regret is not having it sooner. There are infinite ways to find your own path.

Another difficulty I was faced with for the first few weeks was that because of the size of my stomach and all of my stitches, staples, clips, IVs and PICC line, I couldn't even reach to wipe myself when I went to the bathroom. This was an especially embarrassing and troublesome fact for me. If I went to the bathroom, which I did quite frequently, I had to have someone else wipe for me. This task mostly fell to Jeff and my mom. But sometimes, if a friend stayed with me, they might have to wipe for me. I always told them this before they stayed with me, but that didn't ease the sheer humiliation of it all. I tried to keep my sense of humor about it, as did those around me, but the thought of it still makes me cringe today. So, for those unfortunate souls who were close to me during that time, thank you for wiping my butt. I checked at Hallmark, and there weren't any cards that dealt with that situation, so a public thank you, in the middle of my book, will have to suffice, I guess. Somehow it doesn't quite seem like enough, but what more can I say?

This incredibly embarrassing topic does bring up an amazingly beautiful moment of love and courage. When Jeff would go home for the weekend, my mom would take care of me. She would just walk over to my house, stay as long as necessary, and care for Alec and me. On the rare occasions that she needed to go back home for a while, if we needed anything we could call her and she would be right over. At nighttime, she would go home, and if I had to get up and go to the bathroom, I would call her and she would walk over just to wipe for me. Talk about an annoying phone call to receive. On one particular night, I must have gotten up every hour or so with diarrhea. I called her, and she got out of bed, walked over in her nightgown, helped me, and put me back to bed.

Around 4:00 a.m., I woke up and had to go to the

bathroom again. I walked down the hall and had forgotten the cordless phone to call her. Alec heard me in the bathroom, woke up and asked if I needed help. I asked him to please call Grandma and let her know that I needed her again. He called her from the phone in his room, which was right beside the bathroom, and I heard his little voice say, "Grandma, Code Red." This was what he always said to her when I needed her to come help me in the bathroom. I went to the bathroom and I waited, but she never came. This was very unlike her, as she usually came walking in our back door within a few minutes of my call. I waited another ten minutes, and I became concerned. I called out to Alec and asked him to call Grandma back because she never came. He dialed her number and he told me the line was busy.

The next thing I knew my little boy was standing in the bathroom doorway. I can see him to this day. He was barefoot and had on his little red, white, and blue superman underwear and a plain white t-shirt. He announced that he was going to go get Grandma and he'd be right back. Just like that, he was running out the back door of our house, barefoot, in search of help for his mommy. This little boy had to run through our back yard, through my parent's side yard, and around the back of their house to get to my mom's back door. It was 4:00 in the morning and it was pitch black outside. He never thought for one minute that he might be afraid or that he was running into the darkness. He just knew that his mommy needed help and he was going to get it.

Within a few minutes, he came walking into the bathroom holding hands with my mom and smiling from ear to ear. My mom had been so tired that after she answered the phone she fell back asleep. She hadn't even put the phone back in the cradle. She said the next thing she knew this little hand was patting her face saying, "Grandma, Code Red." She was so overwhelmed by the love it took for him, without a second thought, to run into the night, through the darkness, to help his mommy. That amazing little boy of mine put love into action, and to this day, every single time I think of that moment, it moves me to tears.

I also think of all of the care that my mom and Jeff gave to me. My mom was 66 years old at the time and basically cared for me around the clock. Even during the week when Jeff was here to help, my mom was with me every single day, making sure Jeff was taking care of me properly. She drove me to all of my doctor's appointments, did an amazing job taking care of me, and at the same time, still took care of her home and my dad. When I really think about it, at my current age, I don't know that I could have done all that she did and not have been continuously exhausted. I wonder all the time, where in the world did all that strength come from?

As for Jeff, he had his own home that he shared with his girlfriend and her children. He came down, stayed, and took care of me for several weeks, Monday through Friday. He always said that he didn't want anyone else staying with his son, and he wanted his son to know that no matter what happens in life, this is how you treat your mother. He said that he wanted our son to know that even though our relationship didn't work out, it didn't mean we didn't love each other. Love has many faces. It's powerful and sometimes defies reason, but it never disappears and it always shows up. It lasts. It perseveres.

"Love still stands when all else has fallen."

I CORINTHIANS 13:7-10,

CHAPTER 8

"Setting goals is the first step in turning the invisible into the visible"

—Tony Robbins

On the day of my surgery I weighed in at 391 pounds. The charts in my family doctor's office said that I should weigh 165 pounds. I was a long way from that weight. I needed to lose 226 pounds to get to that number. It was simply overwhelming. In my mind, it just seemed like too much to lose. Deep inside of me, even after having the surgery, I doubted that I could do it. In the last 15 years, I hadn't been able to lose any significant amount of weight, so even though I prayed with all my might that I would make it this time, I didn't truly believe I could. I had heard about a lady who had recently lost 80 pounds, and people were so amazed by her huge weight loss. I knew I had to lose almost three times that amount. The negative demons in my mind kept telling me that I could never make it, that it would never really happen.

Why do we have that inner negative voice that speaks to us saying that we can't accomplish the things we truly desire? Why do we have those negative thoughts that tell us we aren't good enough or pretty enough or thin enough? Where do those thoughts and feelings originate? Why do we always first jump to the negative thought instead of the positive thought? Understanding where those thoughts come from allows us to change those patterns of thinking and silence those debilitating and hurtful inner voices. Weren't we all taught in kindergarten that if we don't have anything nice to say, don't say anything at all? Shouldn't we apply that rule to ourselves as well?

People might think we're crazy telling ourselves to shut up, but I don't place too much emphasis on what other people think. After all, I am the Homecoming Queen of Crazy Town. I wear an invisible tiara, a sash, and carry around a Loving Cup that no one else can see. At times, I have shared my reign with nearly all of my friends. The Queen has been an imaginary celebrity in our lives for years. But keep in mind when one is wearing that crown, she is never making the healthy, positive, graceful, mature choice. That is not what the queen is about. I can't tell you how many times a friend of mine, frustrated with a husband, boyfriend, family member, etc., has said, "Girl, give me that crown, because I am about to go act up." While those instances have provided us with some really entertaining stories over the years, they never really ended with any of us getting what we desired. Ever.

In spite of all of the negative thoughts that had become my closest companions over the last decade, somewhere inside of me, there was that inner fire that refused to be extinguished. If I had really given up, I would have never had the surgery. I wouldn't have fought so hard to get it approved and financed. We all have that inner fire. At some points in our lives it may be very faint, and it might just be barely flickering, but it is there, waiting to be fanned into a huge fire providing light and warmth in our lives. At those dim times in our lives, it's crucial to remember Pandora's Box and the last thing to escape from it, hope. Hope is the substance that is like gasoline to that little, tiny flame. Hope ignites our spirit. With hope, what was once a miniscule flame, can explode into a determination and a drive not only to survive, but to thrive and succeed.

In those first several weeks following my surgery, I had to cling to that hope with all I had. I was completely overwhelmed. I was physically weak and exhausted. I was in such bad shape when I came home from the hospital that it took me a couple of months just to be pain free. I didn't have any assistance or comfort from food, which had been my favorite coping mechanism over the last fifteen years. I was on an emotional roller coaster trying to deal with all of my constantly-changing emotions and figure out a new, effective, healthy way to cope.

I tried to think about how wonderful my results were going to be, but I was blinded by all of the immediate physical challenges and difficulties I was currently trying desperately to overcome. Even I didn't realize how much I depended on food to get me through the day. Throughout my life I had been a fan of inspirational quotations. I had always derived major motivation from the written word, and during this difficult time I would pour over my books of quotations looking for some of that same inspiration and guidance. I finally found a beautiful quote by Helen Keller that really struck a chord within my heart. "Optimism is the faith that leads to achievement. Nothing can be done without hope and confidence."

I decided that I needed to think positively. I needed to allow only positive thoughts, feelings, and people into my life. This was a daunting task considering the fact that for many years I had felt so unworthy and inferior. It was also much more difficult to eliminate negative people from my circle than I ever imagined. To be honest, I have only recently discovered not only how essential positive people are to my happiness, but how important it is to be strong enough and have the courage to make that happen. But we all have to crawl before we walk, and I continue to learn as I journey through this life of mine.

I started by thinking positively. I told myself every morning that I could get through the day and that I could do a little more than I did the day before. I would walk all the way out to the kitchen instead of just walking to the bathroom. Each time I went to the bathroom, I then would walk slowly out to the kitchen and then back to the bedroom. It was a very small goal, but it was huge for me. I was still in a lot of pain and still on oxygen. Just walking to the bathroom was hard. But I made myself do it. It was a start.

I also decided to make very small goals for myself so that I could have little successes rather quickly. The scale that I had in my home could only weigh up to 350 pounds. Since I started at 391, I had to lose 41 pounds before I could even weigh myself at home. It was a bit of a blessing that I couldn't weigh myself at home yet, because I was obsessed with how much I weighed. I would have been on that scale morning, noon, and night if it could have weighed me. I desperately needed to see that number going downhill. It reinforced my hope.

Because I am an impatient sort, however, I would get on the scale at home anyway. It was a digital scale, and all it would read was "E." A great big, red, capital "E." The "E" stood for "error," and that just annoyed me as well. When I had a doctor's appointment, I couldn't wait to get on that scale. I was still going to the doctor weekly, and it really did seem as though the weight was melting off of me. No matter how much it was, though, it wasn't enough for me. I simply couldn't lose the weight fast enough. As unrealistic as it was, I wanted to wake up thin. And wearing my tiara, of course.

I still remember the day that I was first able to read my weight on my scale at home. I knew I was getting close to the much awaited 350 pounds, so I was jumping on that scale every morning. Each day when I would see an "E," I would exhale a breathy sigh, accompany it with an even larger eye roll, and walk out of the bathroom. In desperation, I decided to wait a few days before getting back on the scale. When I decided to try again, I turned on the scale, waited for the bright red double zeroes to appear, and stepped up. I waited the second or two that it took to register. This time, instead of an "E," it read 348. I was so happy and so excited, I must have gotten off and on that thing ten times, making sure it read 348 each time.

My celebration was short-lived, though. Soon, those negative feelings, derived from all those years of low self-esteem, began to infiltrate and darken what was a happy, light, joy-filled moment. Instead of being proud of myself, I wondered what kind of woman celebrates weighing 348 pounds? I'm still a fat cow. I'm still huge to the rest of the world. It must be really pathetic to celebrate weighing 348 pounds. I shared these feelings with both my mom and Lori, who were quick to tell me that I couldn't think that way and that I should be proud of myself. I can remember Lori's words: "Don't be so hard on yourself, you're doing great, and I'm really proud of you." My mom's sentiment was pretty much the same, but her delivery was a little different. It started with "Kelley Elizabeth…" and ended with her talking to Jesus, Mary, and Joseph again. In the course of my lifetime, she talked to that trio quite a bit.

I'm not certain why I let those negative thoughts creep into my mind and try to destroy my new happiness. I have a

Master's Degree in counseling, for goodness sake. I knew that thinking those negative thoughts was very self-defeating, but I just couldn't completely extinguish them. As I would discover many years down the road, those thoughts didn't originate from my weight or my body image. No matter how much weight I lost or how I looked, until I figured that emotional complexity out, I was going to continue to struggle with all of that negativity deep inside my soul. That quiet beast, the monster who was hidden from almost everyone who knew me, would take years to slay.

My next goal after hitting 348 was to get to 320. As complicated as this thought seems, I couldn't wait to weigh 319 and be able to say that I only had 19 pounds to lose until my weight never started with a three again. Believe it or not, I actually hit 299 within three months of my surgery. I lost 91 pounds in the first 90 days. I was so excited to finally start with a two. But again, my negative thoughts kicked in, and I chastised myself for being excited to weigh 299 pounds. When I reached 291 and I could say that I had lost 100 pounds, even that happiness was short lived because I thought that only a lunatic would be happy to weigh 291 pounds. I thought, "Don't kid yourself. The world still sees you as a 300-pound woman, and no one finds that attractive." My brain was in an argument with my soul on a daily basis.

My happy and proud soul was fighting for its right to be proud of its accomplishment. The nasty little dictator who had been in charge of all that low self-esteem and negative thinking was not going down so easily. That emotional dictator had been in charge of my thoughts and feelings for my entire life. It wasn't going to relinquish its power so quickly. For as long as I could remember, I had fought for joy and happiness. I was always a happy person on the outside, appearing to others as bubbly and joy-filled. In those quiet alone moments, though, I knew I wasn't enough. I knew I needed to be better. No matter what I accomplished, it was never enough.

This sense of inadequacy had always been an issue for me. In high school I had been voted Student of the Quarter and it was published in the local paper. I remember reading it and thinking that I hadn't done enough and didn't deserve the award. I knew I wasn't as good as anyone else. I knew I couldn't let anyone else close enough to me, or they would discover my truth: I wasn't good enough.

In spite of all the internal emotional battles, however, the happy, positive side of me was gaining momentum. It was as though it was being fed Miracle-Gro of the soul. Happy thoughts and hopeful desires were beginning to become stronger and stronger and take over my thoughts. Of course, negativity would still pop up, but I could push it out of my mind more quickly than before.

There is a weight loss "window" for my type of surgery, which lasts roughly 18-24 months. During this time, the surgically-reduced stomach begins to stretch and patients can begin to eat a little more than in the beginning. So, people who have undergone the surgery need to strive to lose all the weight they can during those first 18 months. Dr. Maguire had told me to limit my sugar intake to a certain amount each day. I stuck to that amount religiously. Sugar was the one substance that I would absorb completely, and I took that seriously. Unfortunately, sugar had been, and always will be, my weakness. But I was determined to make my goal weight during the first 18 months, and so I avoided sugar like the plague. For Christmas that year Lori brought over a plate of her wonderful homemade Christmas cookies, and I remember wanting a cookie so desperately. I sat there and argued with myself about a cookie. This was the fifth month since my surgery and I hadn't even had a bite of a cookie yet. I decided to make myself a deal. I ate half a cookie.

One might think that after all this time, the cookie probably didn't taste as good as I remembered. Well, I'm here to tell you that cookie, in short, tasted like Heaven. That cookie had *me* talking to Jesus, Mary and Joseph. Luckily for me, I had that little son of mine, who had recently turned eight, and he was more than happy to destroy that plate of cookies within no time at all, so I wasn't tempted to eat any more of them. In fact, as he grabbed the plate to disappear into the room with Lori's daughters, he announced that it was the least he could do.

Whether this is a blessing or a curse, I still love sugar to this day. I have never done drugs in my life, but if sugar were a drug, it would be my crack. It remains my weakness. Lori, who is still my best friend, shares my desire to find the best baked goods in the world. It's a mission we take rather seriously. Today, I still indulge from time to time, but I've just learned to do so in a much more mediated fashion. I told myself during my weight loss that I could put off sugar for 18 months if it meant that I could reach my goal weight. I reminded myself daily that I didn't have to live without it forever, just for a while, so that I could reach my goal quicker. My belief then, and my belief today, is that life is too short not to enjoy the things you love. Moderation is the key.

Hear me when I tell you, though, sometimes I have fallen off the wagon and have gone buck wild. I am not perfect and will never claim to be. During those times, I have to have a talk with myself and say, "Okay crack baby, enough! Get back to healthy." But by and large, my attitude in life is that it is important to enjoy the things you love and to realize that we are all here only for a spell. As Erma Bombeck said, "Seize the moment. Remember all those women on the *Titanic* who waved off the *dessert cart*." When it comes to food, I try to make two to three healthy choices for each unhealthy choice I make. Sometimes I lose that battle, and sometimes I win. It's really about finding a method that works for you.

Making small goals may not work for everyone, but it worked well for me. It still does. When I reached 288 pounds,

I made my next goal getting to 280. I would think that I only had nine more pounds until I was in a new ten's digit. That kept my goals short, and I was able to reach them relatively quickly. Everyone close to me knew my method and would ask me how many more pounds I had to lose until I was in a new ten's digit.

The weight continued to melt away. I ate right, I drank all of the water I was supposed to, and I took my vitamins. I also exercised. Exercise was so difficult for me initially, so in the beginning I didn't do much. As I began to lose weight, though, things got a little easier for me. In the beginning, simply walking was a major victory for me. It had been so hard for me to walk anywhere, and now I could walk and not be short of breath so quickly. When I had reached 300 pounds, I decided I would start another form of exercise. I spoke to a trainer at the local YMCA and was told that water aerobics or swimming might be good for me because it wouldn't be as hard on my joints and body as any other type of aerobic activity. I still weighed 300 pounds, and most exercise was going to be incredibly hard on my body. I also didn't really want to be in the middle of a workout room with other, potentially critical people, so I wanted to choose something that was a little more private for me. The trainer told me that their water aerobics class started at 7:00 a.m., and most of the people in the class were retired, older women, so that seemed like a good choice for me.

My soul felt a little safer within this group of people, and

I felt like the chances of my being ridiculed were minimal. Because I was a single mom, I had to sign my son up for the class as well. I couldn't leave him home alone. His school didn't start until 8:55 a.m., so he could go to the 50-minute class with me, and I could still have him showered and to school by 8:55 since the YMCA was only five minutes from our home. He absolutely loved the class. The older, retired ladies who were my new workout partners were a bit surprised when he came charging out of the locker room yelling, "CANNON-BALL!" and jumped into the middle of the pool, but the class and the people were wonderful, and it really worked for me.

As a result of being at the YMCA, I would also swim laps after the class. I wasn't strong enough to swim anything but the backstroke at the time, but I would do as many laps as I could, and each day I would try to add a lap or two. Eventually I asked the lifeguard how many laps made a mile, and he informed me it was 75 laps. I could only swim about 18 laps at the time. But I made it my goal to work my way up to swimming a mile. I would drop Alec off at school and go back and swim laps. It took me a couple of months, but I eventually could swim a mile, doing the backstroke. The lifeguard even added my name to their "Mile Book."

I was very proud of my swimming, and the water aerobics really helped in my weight loss. I was losing even more quickly because of the extra activity. After a few months of this, however, I was at school one day speaking with Alec's teacher.

She was asking about my weight loss, as she had been a very positive supporter from the beginning. I told her that we had been doing water aerobics every morning, and she said, "Oh… so that's why Alec is falling asleep every afternoon in class." So that was the end of water aerobics. I would have to find another way to exercise because I couldn't have my son falling asleep in class.

Needless to say, because I was losing so much weight so quickly, I was going through major wardrobe changes faster than you can imagine. In the beginning, almost all of the clothes I had were too small for me and tight anyway. I was a size 32, but I also had many smaller-sized outfits in my closet that I had outgrown along the way. At first it was so exciting because things became too big for me very quickly, and getting into old outfits felt wonderful.

Specifically, I can remember one particular outfit that I had received for Christmas one year. It was still in my closet with the tags on it because I had been too embarrassed to tell the person who gave it to me that it was way too small. At one point after losing weight, I had tried it on and it was still too small, so I forgot about it for a while. When I remembered it again, I couldn't wait to get it out and try it on. When I tried it on the second time, I had lost so much weight so quickly that it was already too big for me to wear. I felt disappointed for a second, and then reminded myself that this was actually a pretty fantastic disappointment. What an amazing oxymoron!

It actually became somewhat expensive to keep clothes in my closet that fit. I had to work, and I needed clothes to wear that fit me appropriately. I began buying just a couple of pairs of pants that fit me, mixing and matching several shirts to go along with them. I just couldn't afford to buy new clothes as quickly as I needed them, so I did the best I could. Still, this was a blessing in disguise, and was one inconvenience I embraced. It also made it quite easy for my friends and family to know what to give me as a gift.

As I continued to lose more and more weight, I remembered that when friends used to tell me that they needed to lose 30 or 40 pounds, I would always think to myself that if I only needed to lose 30 or 40 pounds, I wouldn't even bother losing it. When you need to lose 240 pounds, being overweight by 30 or 40 pounds seems like a walk in the park. I felt that I could easily be happy at 30 or 40 pounds overweight.

It's so easy to compare ourselves to other people and think we could be happier in their situation. As humans, we constantly are guilty of thinking that the grass is greener on the other side. We never stop to think that the grass, wherever it is and however green it is, still has to be mowed. No one has a beautiful lawn without taking care of it. All kinds of nasty and poisonous things that you don't want in your yard can pop up in there if you don't treat it correctly. It's the same with our bodies, minds, and souls. We have to take care of those things constantly and provide them with the positive components needed to stay healthy and to allow us to thrive on all levels. We have to be always willing to pull the weeds out of our lives or they will take it over, just like crab grass in a yard.

I hadn't taken care of me in a long time. I hadn't taken care of myself physically, spiritually, or emotionally. Now, as I was beginning to lose weight and evolve into something new, all of the parts of my being were being challenged and changed. Positive changes in our lives are just as stressful as negative ones. It's a ripple effect. It's basically Newton's third law, "For every action, there is an equal and opposite reaction." As I lost weight and changed, so did every situation and every person around me.

This change was something for which I was unprepared. When people had discouraged me from having the surgery, I didn't really put a lot of thought into why they would feel that way. They always prefaced their arguments with statements professing that they loved me and they were worried about me and they thought the surgery could be dangerous. My intuitive nature naturally sensed that something was not right with these arguments from these particular individuals, but I pushed those thoughts down into that place I didn't visit regularly.

Some of my family members would mention health concerns, and I genuinely knew they were concerned as to the safety of the surgery. But once I had shared all of the information with my family members, they felt comfortable as to the safety of the surgery. In contrast, the other individuals would still vocalize their opinions, some rather harshly, along with their displeasure that I was going to go through with the surgery. This is when I truly began to learn that sometimes, weak and insecure people build their image of themselves based on their perception of you. If you change, then their perception of you changes, and that will alter their image of themselves.

Some of my friends had weight issues themselves, but without a doubt I was by far the heaviest person in my entire circle of friends. It never crossed my mind that my friends who had their own weight issues felt better about themselves when compared to me. Later, I found out from others that some of these friends would make comments in reference to my weight and say things like, "I would **never** let myself get as big as Kelley. I would starve myself first," or "I realize I'm big, but Kelley is HUGE," or "When I'm at an event and I want to make sure no one thinks I've gained weight, I just stand by Kelley."

Initially hearing those things really hurt my feelings, but I have learned that those comments really had nothing to do with me at all. These people already felt bad about themselves and were simply looking for any comparison to make themselves feel better. So, of course when I decided to have a surgery that would finally give me the opportunity to lose a large amount of weight, the thought of me changing who

I was became very threatening to them. They were safe and secure with Fat Kelley. Fat Kelley wasn't a threat to anyone. If she changed and lost weight, that would change their perception of everything, including themselves. It would force them to have to look at who and what they truly were. They would lose the empty ego game in which they always came out the winner by comparison. That was scary for them. The hardest thing in the world is to look at the true picture of who we are without any filters.

The game of self-deceit is a tricky, multi-faceted one. I don't believe that any of those friends were acutely aware of how they felt. I don't believe for a second that they thought that my being fat made them feel better. I also don't believe that they were capable of the introspection that it takes to realize what made them feel that way. I don't know that they could even admit that they felt that way.

On a positive note, I have to say that not all of my friends with weight issues were insecure at all and not all of them felt negatively toward my situation. A few of them were among my biggest supporters and cheered me on every step of the way. At the time, as an insecure person myself, I focused more of my attention on the negative people. Their voices were always louder than the positive people. This is because I was always trying to earn everyone's approval. Their acceptance made me feel better about myself. I didn't have the confidence to stand firm in my decision on my own.

Thank God for Lori because she was all the backbone I needed. She constantly defended my decision both to me and to others. Whenever I would be upset over something someone had said and start doubting that I was doing the right thing, she would remind me of all of the reasons this was the right decision for me. She would also remind me in no uncertain terms that this was no one else's business. Once my Mom was on board with me having the surgery, she was also a staunch defender of my decision. When I would become upset about my friends who disapproved of my decision to have the surgery, my mom would constantly tell me, "Stop putting your wishbone where your backbone should be. You made this decision, now stand by it."

The truth is, the decisions we make to improve our lives cause others to look at their own. If they're doing nothing to improve their own lives and are unhappy, they will be uncomfortable with our decision to fight for something better. It's the perfect example of the butterfly effect, which is defined by Merriam-Webster as, "a property of chaotic systems (such as the atmosphere) by which small changes in initial conditions can lead to large-scale and unpredictable variation in the future state of the system." To simplify, any behavior and change of our own starts a ripple effect into the lives of everyone else we know. The word "unpredictable" jumps out at me here because I can honestly say that I could have never predicted some of the changes in the people around me. More surprising than the changes themselves, were the people who changed. Another lesson I have learned in life is that people will always surprise you. They will surprise you in both good ways and in bad ways. There is no predicting it, and there is no getting around that fact.

After I had lost around 100 pounds, one of my closest friends was talking with me on the phone. She had a weight problem of her own and probably needed to lose about 90 pounds. I still had roughly 143 pounds to lose, and we were discussing the day's events when suddenly she randomly said, "When you get smaller than me, that's when we're going to have a problem." Then she laughed and said she was just kidding. It was awkward and almost eerie. Since high school I have been well-aware of the fact that the truth is often clothed in jest. I knew at the time that she meant it, laugh or no laugh. Throughout my weight-loss journey, I would come to find out that difficulties in personal friendships would be all too common in my new existence, but it was all part of my complex journey of growth and change.

I was always taught by both my mom and my Nonnie that without change, growth cannot occur. As fast as I was losing weight, I was growing as a person, but that growth wasn't easy, and it wasn't always the result of anything positive. Eventually I was faced with the hard, cold, reality that I was going to lose some people I had thought were my friends. It was a pretty hard pill for me to swallow. At the time, I just couldn't understand how anyone couldn't be happy for me. If the situation were reversed, I felt I would have been happy for them. But I've slowly accepted that not everyone is capable of that, because they lack the self-confidence to feel secure in someone else's success. Slowly, some people begin to realize that they are no longer comfortable in your presence because your improvements make them focus on the things they don't like about themselves. Needless to say, that doesn't feel very good. When that happens, those people have a tendency to redirect the blame with accusations, or by distancing themselves.

These negative people probably don't even realize what they are actually feeling. People would tell me I had changed. And they were right, I had. But they would say that I was arrogant or simply make up a reason for why they just didn't want to be around me anymore. Some people might call this jealousy, but I think it's deeper than that. I would call it a discomfort with self, an unacceptance, and a lack of love for who they are.

Looking back, I remember that Dr. Maguire had said that I was going to lose some people along the way and that some of them might be surprising. He told me that I needed to prepare myself for that fact. At the time, I really didn't think that would happen to me. I didn't think I would lose anyone simply because I lost weight. I was wrong.

When I was growing up, my mom always told me, "Pay very close attention to who doesn't clap when you win." I used to get so tired of hearing that from her. I finally have been able to absorb the truth in that age-old message. Jealousy is a very unhealthy, negative force. It's powerful, and if fed, it destroys what is wonderful and good. Jealousy can cause healthy people to think and act in very unhealthy ways. Jealousy truly is an illness, and while we can pray that many people out there get well soon, we can't delay our own happiness waiting for that to happen.

People who love you will want you to shine, plain and simple. A couple years ago, I attended a week-long educational seminar that addressed how we form attachments and bond to others. While the entire event was quite interesting and educational, one thing the doctor presented really caught my soul's attention. In order to be able truly to love someone, we need to feel safe to shine in their presence. He wasn't referring necessarily to romantic love, but to all the different kinds of love. This really hit home for me and made me think of Nonnie, who always told me, "Never dim your light for anybody, baby." I had done just that, though. I had always been afraid to do something better than someone else because I didn't want them to stop liking me.

In high school I can remember lying to a friend about my score on a test, because I didn't want her to be angry that I did better than her. Many times throughout my career I wouldn't be forthcoming about an evaluation or praise from my supervisor, because I wouldn't want my co-workers to be angry. As I recall that now, I'm saddened that I ever felt that

I had to lessen who I was to win the approval of others. So many things fell into place for me emotionally when I heard the doctor's words. If you don't feel safe to shine in someone's presence, you will never have the true connection with them that healthy love should allow.

The reality of it remains that when you change yourself, all of the people around you will change as well. Some of those changes will be positive and, sadly, some will be negative and hurtful. This fact can't stop you from becoming all you are meant to be. Another thing Nonnie told me many times while I was growing up was, "Blowing out someone else's candle doesn't make yours shine any brighter." It takes a pretty wise person to know that, and an incredibly confident person to live their life with that as their mantra. Always remember that you have the absolute God-given right to shine your fullest, brightest light out into the world. In fact, it is your responsibility to do so.

"You playing small doesn't serve the world. There's nothing enlightening about shrinking so others won't feel insecure around you. As you let your own light shine, you indirectly give others permission to do the same."

—Marianne Williamson

CHAPTER 9

"God will command his angels to protect you wherever you go."

PSALM 91:11

AS TIME PASSED, so did most of the physical difficulties associated with my surgery. As the months went by, I experienced fewer negative side effects and more positive ones. Within a few months, I felt so much better and had so much more energy that I was amazed by the things I was starting to be able to do. I could walk to my parent's house next door and not need to stop for a break or to catch my breath. The smallest things that would be insignificant to other people were reasons for me to celebrate.

The first time I carried my own groceries inside and didn't need help, I actually thanked God. There had been a time when even going to the grocery was a struggle for me. I literally had to use the grocery cart to hold me up while walking through the store. I would have to bend over the cart all the time because my back hurt so much. When I would finish paying for my items, I would call my mom, and she would meet me at my house and carry my groceries in for me, because I couldn't do it. I was thrilled to declare that those days were behind me.

The one negative side effect that continued longer than I would have liked was the vomiting. I must have vomited daily for about eight or nine months. The other patients I spoke with at the support group had that problem initially, but it dissipated for them much more quickly than mine did. I had a stalker, and he lived in my stomach. That little man with his trampoline did not want to leave me. Eventually, though, he did finally go on his way, and around ten months after my surgery, the daily vomiting stopped.

A lot had happened around me during those months. My son had breezed through the second grade. He had been blessed with an amazing teacher, Mrs. Dowd. At Kyle Elementary where he attended, the first and second grade teacher "looped," which meant that he had Mrs. Dowd for both the first and the second grade. He adored her. He soaked up every bit of wisdom that she gave him and luckily, she was an amazing human being. She was loaded with spirit and spark and was one of the most bubbly and happy people I have ever known. She was kindness personified but she also had a backbone of steel and didn't let those children push her around one bit.

I suppose that strength and inner beauty is what allowed her to be such a huge support to me, someone that she barely knew. My surgery had taken place in August between Alec's first and second grade years. So as the school year progressed and I continued to lose weight, Mrs. Dowd was one of my biggest cheerleaders. She would sing my praises and offer me more encouragement than I could have ever expected. She genuinely was happy for me. In May, ten months after my surgery, I had gone to school for something and she grabbed me by the hand and pulled me into her classroom. She stood me up in front of the entire class and told them all how much weight I had lost and had them all clap for me. It made me smile from ear-to-ear to have a room full of second graders applauding and cheering for me. Of course, my son was leading the cheers, and it warmed my heart to see how happy and proud he was.

As I've mentioned, there were several angels I encountered throughout this journey, and Ginny Dowd was definitely one of them. The first time I ever saw her I thought how I would give anything to trade places with her. She was petite, thin, and beautiful. She was simply alive and so full of life. She was like a magnet, and everyone wanted to be close to her. She seemed to ooze positivity out of her pores. I desperately wanted to be that kind of person. She only knew me as a parent of one of the children in her class, yet she provided me with encouragement and hope. She touched and changed my life in a way that she will never know. I believe those people are sprinkled throughout our journey to reinforce that we are on the right track. Those special, unexpected moments of praise are the universe's way of acknowledging our efforts. The journey of a huge weight loss is a long one and along the way, we need those surprise celebrations to inspire us to keep going. Sometimes the support of someone who isn't family or a part of our inner circle, makes all the difference in the world.

In May, my surgery was ten months behind me. I had lost 186 pounds and weighed 205. I was so excited because I was taking my very first vacation with my little boy. Prior to this, I wouldn't have been able to travel for many reasons. First, I couldn't fit in an airplane seat, and I was horrified at the thought of having to get an extender or purchase two seats because of my size. I couldn't afford first class, where the seats were bigger, and I couldn't afford to purchase two seats just for me. Second, even if I could have figured out the traveling, once we got to our destination, I couldn't have done anything because I couldn't walk anywhere. So, this first vacation for my son and me was a very big deal. He was getting out of school at the end of May, and we were leaving for Orlando, Florida, and Universal Studios the very next day. My son was so excited, he couldn't sleep the night before. He had been waiting to get to Jurassic Park for as long as he could remember.

Every day we received a new brochure in the mail from Universal Studios, detailing some amazing new attraction. Alec ran to the mailbox daily to grab anything new that might have arrived.

The day before we were leaving, he came trotting through the kitchen with the mail in his hands, and threw an envelope on the counter, announcing that nothing good had come.

Chuckling to myself, I walked over and picked up the mail. It was a letter from my insurance company. I opened it, expecting it to be an explanation of benefits from one of my many ongoing office visits with Dr. Maguire. But, it wasn't. It was an explanation of benefits to Kettering Hospital. I assumed it was for lab work or one of the many other tests I had done there regularly. But to my amazement, I quickly realized it was a statement detailing that the insurance company had approved my third appeal and had reimbursed Kettering Hospital for every cent of my surgical cost. It had been several months since I had submitted my third appeal and I had completely forgotten about it. The first two were denied so quickly, I had assumed this one was rejected as well.

It took a few moments for the full reality to sink in. Suddenly it hit me. I had won my appeal! My insurance had paid my entire hospital bill, and that meant I was going to get reimbursed every dollar that I had paid Kettering Hospital for my surgery. I immediately fell onto my knees and began praying and thanking God. After all of the struggles I encountered trying to obtain the finances for my surgery, now I was getting all of that money reimbursed. I simply couldn't thank God long enough or loud enough. I was overwhelmed with gratitude and happiness.

A very curious Alec came running into the kitchen to investigate the source of my joyful screams. We celebrated together and did our little version of the happy dance. He gave me a big hug, and announced that now, since we had a little extra money, we could purchase a dinosaur at Jurassic Park during our vacation.

I was so excited with life at the time. I weighed 205 pounds, and that meant that I only had FIVE pounds to go until I no longer started with the number two. This was a momentous event for me. I hadn't started with a one in over 15 years. I couldn't even remember how my body felt the last time my weight started with a one. I couldn't remember how it felt when I weighed 199. It didn't really matter anymore what I used to feel like, because I was currently feeling the best I'd felt in nearly two decades. Having said that, I simply couldn't wait to finally weigh in under 200 pounds.

I read at the time that most people gain five pounds when they are on vacation. I did NOT want that to happen to me. I lost sleep thinking about that. I also wanted to be able to enjoy my vacation, though, and try some of the amazing meals and desserts that were shown on the commercials and the videos we had watched. I decided that I would try my best to maintain my weight at 205 during our trip. I wouldn't deprive myself while I was there, but I also wouldn't go too far off my eating plan. I planned that Alec and I could order one of the amazing desserts we saw on TV and we could share it. I thought that even if I just had a couple of bites, at least I would get to try it and share the experience with my son. What I didn't plan on, was that my life was about to change forever.

Universal Studios say in their commercials that a vacation there is the adventure of a lifetime. For us, that was an understatement. Neither my son nor I would ever be the same. People speak of having a once-in-a-lifetime moment, but who knew mine was going to be at a theme park in Orlando, Florida?

The big day finally arrived, and as we boarded the plane I still thought, "Will I be able to fit in the seat?" My heart was racing, and I had a severe feeling of panic as I sat down in the seat. It didn't matter that I had lost 186 pounds; that fear, that humiliation and shame, that panic of, "What do I do if I don't fit into this seat," was overwhelming to me. I felt that everyone's eyes were on me as I successfully strapped myself into the seat, when in fact, not a single person was paying a bit of attention. I was able to forget about my own insecurities and fears when I remembered that Alec had never flown, and this was a huge deal for him. He was so thrilled, and his eyes were dancing with excitement. He held my hand as we took off, and when we reached cruising, he looked at me and said, "That was AMAZING!"

We arrived in Orlando. Since we were staying at the Hard Rock Hotel, our room key was also our pass to get into the Universal Studios theme parks all week. As you can imagine, we were off and running within five minutes of checking into our room. The first two days went by without a hitch. We went to Universal Studios and enjoyed the attractions and ate at all of the amazing restaurants. Eating in an appropriate fashion wasn't nearly the difficult scenario that I had envisioned it being. I ordered dessert and shared it with Alec and only ate a bite or two. I was proud of the restraint I showed and I didn't feel deprived on any level. Plus, we walked and walked and walked. I was getting a lot more exercise than I did at home, so even if I did have more calories than usual, I thought it should all even out.

On the third day, we were back at Universal Studios and in line for the Back to the Future ride. An interesting thing about Universal is that all of the line areas are themed according to the attraction you are waiting to ride. We had just gotten into the final room before boarding the ride. Suddenly, I was very dizzy and the room started spinning. The sounds around me started to sound far away and as if I were in a barrel. I looked at Alec and told him I didn't feel well. I had experienced these same symptoms once before while we were grocery shopping, and I recognized them immediately. I knew I was about to pass out. I told Alec that Mommy needed help and I leaned up against a wall as everything began to fade to black.

The next thing I knew, I was sitting on a bench outside of the ride and one of the employees told me that they had called for the medics. Immediately I was worried about Alec and asked where my son was. I heard Alec say, "I'm right here Mommy. Please don't be mad at me for coming outside alone, but I had to walk out here and get help because none of the people inside the room would help me." I told him I wasn't mad at him at all, but asked what he meant when he said no one would help him. He explained that when I fainted, he told the people in the room that his mommy needed help, and they all just looked at him and did nothing.

At that point, he ran out of the room and went to the outside waiting area and told an employee his mommy needed help. They had come inside the room, found me on the floor, and helped me to a bench outside the attraction. The employee instructed me to sit with my elbows on my knees and to keep my head down. While waiting on the medics to arrive, an incredibly kind gentleman walked up beside me and reminded me to keep my head down and to rest. I didn't see his face, but I could tell from his voice that he was older. He spoke to me and had an accent that I didn't recognize. He rubbed my back and told me that everything would be okay. I again informed him that I was worried about my son, and he told me that Alec was right there, a few feet away from me, and that his wife was sitting with him and he was fine. I was crying and very worried. This kind stranger continued to tell me that I had no reason to worry.

This man spoke to his wife in a language I didn't recognize and continued to tell me that Alec was right beside me and that we both were in good hands. His wife spoke back to him in the same language. I never did hear her speak English, although her husband spoke it perfectly. I realized at that moment that even though I felt terrible, I wasn't afraid. This man had an incredible presence, and all of my fear completely dissipated. I was, however, crying and I explained to this older gentleman that no one would help my son. I expressed my frustration and asked him how anyone could ignore a little boy in that situation. He let me know that we were not alone, that Alec was never in danger, and that we had all the help we needed.

I was thankful for the compassion and genuine kindness this man and his wife were showing us, but I still was very angry at the people in that line. I couldn't comprehend ignoring a little boy's pleas for help for his mom. As I sat there with my head down and my elbows on my knees, I stared at this kind man's shoes. He was wearing bluish gray Nikes. I thanked him over and over and told him how much it meant to me that he was there and that his wife was sitting with and watching Alec. My mind was racing with worry of what would happen to my son if I had to go to the emergency room, but suddenly, the man told me to stop worrying and that everything would be fine. It was as if he could read my mind.

Suddenly the medics arrived and there was a flurry of activity around me. The medics were firing questions at me left and right, and in the flurry of activity around me, I didn't get to tell the kind man and his wife a final thank you. I raised my head and looked around for them, and realized I didn't even know what they looked like because I'd kept my head down and all I'd seen was his shoes. I asked the medics if they could please point out the gentleman and his wife who took care of us because I wanted to tell them thank you. The medics seemed confused, and I explained that I didn't see their faces but that the man was wearing those blue sneakers. I was immediately looking at the feet of all the people around me, searching for those shoes.

The medics started to push me away toward the on-site clinic, and I told them they had to stop because before I went anywhere I had to thank the kind couple who had helped us so much. The medic looked at me with a bewildered expression and asked who I was referring to. I explained the story again to him. I told him no one else would help us and that they made all the difference in the world. The man looked me straight in my eye and said, "Ma'am, you were alone when we got here."

Incredibly frustrated at this point, I told him that the man and his wife were right here with us. I looked for my son and I said to him, "Baby, where is the nice lady who sat with you and the man who was with me and talking to me the entire time? The couple who were speaking the different language? Where did they walk to? The man who was wearing the bluish gray Nikes, where did he go? Mommy needs to tell them thank you." Alec looked at me with his huge brown eyes and said, "Mommy, we were alone." Immediately I argued the point. My son told me again, "Mommy we were alone the entire time."

With that, the medics whisked me off to their clinic. I continued to insist that there was someone with us the entire time. I couldn't let it go. I knew what I knew and what I knew was, we were not alone. At that point, it occurred to me that we were visited by angels. In the middle of the hustle and bustle of Universal Studios, two angels watched over my son and me until help arrived. It all began to make sense to me. The language was so different than anything I had ever heard. Not that I'm a linguist, but it just seemed distinctively different. To this day, I've never heard anything that even remotely resembled what I heard that day. The calming effect the man had on me had been overwhelming. I just couldn't get over the fact that to everyone walking by us, we appeared alone, but we were far from alone. The strongest power in the Universe had sent us help. How does one react when they realize they have just had an encounter with an actual angel?

I can tell you how I responded. I began sobbing and sobbing. I was overcome. It was perfect validation. I had always believed in God and had always prayed to and loved God. But this was a physical proof that everything I had ever believed in and had faith in was completely true. It was absolutely overwhelming in a beautiful way. To this day I cannot tell that story and not be emotionally overcome. I get chills up and down my spine, goosebumps everywhere, and I am immediately moved to tears. In fact, when I share that story with people, they always seem to have the exact same reaction. It's an amazing revelation to realize that you have actually been touched by an angel. How does anyone ever carry on with their life after an experience such as this and not be forever changed? My strength and inner resolve to finish my weight loss was given a huge boost and I felt as though nothing could stop me. Any doubts I had ever had about having the surgery were removed. My angelic experience provided a firm confirmation that I had made the right choice.

As I have moved forward in my life, I have always been keenly aware that God exists. There have been times when I have been upset with God and disappointed in the events that have happened in my life. I could never get upset enough, though, not to believe in Him. In my mind, I have absolute proof that there are angels, and if there are angels, there is definitely a God. I may become dismayed and lost from time to time, and I may not understand why things are happening or not happening, but what I know for sure is that there is most definitely a God. He sent angels to protect us and if He wanted to protect us, then it's because He has a plan for us. That day, in Orlando, Florida, God dispatched two of his own to wrap their arms around us and keep us safe in their care.

In my darkest, scariest hours, when I start to lose my faith and begin to question everything, eventually my mind travels back to Orlando, Florida and I remember who protected my son and me, and who sent them to do so. In that moment, I realize that even though it seems unclear to me at the time, there is a plan. I can't turn my back on God, because he has proven to me that he is there, and that is something I will never forget. My life certainly hasn't been easy. I have made my share of mistakes, and in no way am I perfect. The one thing I have absolutely no doubt about, though, is that God is perfect and in spite of my errors along the way, He loves me.

My angel encounter provided me with much inner peace as my weight loss continued. In those moments of self-doubt, that would still surface many times in my life, I would reflect on what happened in Orlando and find the strength I needed to carry on. We all find our personal inspiration and motivation in many different ways, and we draw on that in times of hardship. I derive my strength from my faith in God. Yes, God exists, as do angels. I've heard them, had a conversation with one, been touched by them, and one of them wears bluish-gray Nikes.

While my mind was still spinning about my angel encounter, the medics were taking my blood pressure. It was 80 over 40. I explained to them that I had recently had bariatric surgery in the last year and that I carried a laminated card with my surgeon's contact information. Dr. Maguire had always told us that no other physician should treat us without conferring with him first. I gave them the card, which I carried under my driver's license, and they called his office. Of course, the third angel of the day took the phone call. As you can guess, that would be Kim. They explained my condition to her and she spoke with Dr. Maguire. After all of the professionals collaborated, they decided that I had become dehydrated. With all of the excitement of vacation and all of the walking in the heat, I hadn't been careful to keep track of how much water I had drunk over the last three days. Which, when I thought about it, was very little.

Dr. Maguire recommended I go to the emergency room and get fluids to rehydrate me quickly. I didn't want to do that because I was worried about what would happen to my son while I was in the emergency room. I opted to go back to our hotel room and stay in for the rest of the day and also the next day and drink as much water as I possibly could to rehydrate myself. As luck would have it, my cousin Missy lived only a few hours away. I called her, and she took some vacation time to come and stay with Alec and me for the next couple of days.

Universal Studios was wonderful. They not only made sure that I was safely transported back to my hotel, but they extended our stay by two days without charging us any additional fees, so that we wouldn't lose the two days it would take for me to recover. They called to check on us several times over the next two days, and offered to bring food to our rooms or any items that we needed. They were extremely good to us, and they didn't even know about the angels. It's nice to know that a huge corporation like Universal Studios cared about a single mom and her eight-year-old, son from Troy, Ohio. We enjoyed the remainder of our vacation and returned home to Troy with amazing, life-changing memories.

When we arrived home, I simply couldn't wait to get on the scales the next morning. We had originally scheduled seven vacation days, but because of the unexpected extension, it had been almost ten days since I weighed myself. I was so hopeful that I would have maintained my weight and not gained those typical five pounds. I didn't want my much-anticipated goal of getting below two hundred pounds to be delayed any longer than it already had been.

I prepared myself though, because I had ordered dessert every single night at dinner, and I had also indulged in a few treats during the day as well. I only drank water, but I was still worried because I hadn't really eaten any sugar for almost ten months, with the exception of that delicious half-cookie at Christmas. Getting weighed was such an emotional event for me, that I even considered putting it off for a week. I was worried that if I actually gained a pound or two, I would have a total meltdown. I thought it might be smarter to wait until I had been home and back on my strict regimen of no sugar and regular exercise before I stepped on that scale. I must admit, though, I did not possess that level of self-control. For the last ten months, even though Kim and Dr. Maguire both had told me not to weigh myself every single day, I still did. Every morning I would get on that scale. I simply couldn't stand it.

So, on this day, I was no different. I walked into the bathroom and I looked down at my old nemesis, Mr. Scale. I talked to him that day. I explained to him that unless he wanted to take a flying trip out of Mr. Window, he needed to be kind. I looked at myself in the mirror and said, "Kelley, you are standing here talking to a battery operated, digital device and threatening it with a trip out the window if it doesn't display a weight you are comfortable with…you really have reached a whole new level of crazy." Honestly, I was okay with that.

I guess I should mention that I always weighed myself completely naked. I didn't want so much as a single ounce of extra weight from pajamas or any other clothing adding to my weight. So, I ripped off my nightgown and held my breath. I pushed on the scale and waited for it to register double zero so that I could climb on. Two bright red zeros flashed up at me and I stepped onto the scale. I silently said a prayer and waited for the crucial number. I looked down at the scale and almost had a heart attack. It read a very clear, very distinctive, bright red, 196 pounds. I couldn't even believe my eyes. I was in shock. The number on the scale literally took my breath away. I quickly got off the scale and waited on the numbers to turn off. As soon as it was dark, I pushed on it and waited for the double zero to again appear. Immediately, I climbed back onto the scale. I had to see if the weight was correct and if I read it correctly. It again said 196. It didn't say 196.8 or 196.4, it said 196. Not only did I not gain any weight while I was on vacation, but I lost 9 pounds.

I just stood on the scale and looked at the number. The numbers began to appear blurry, and I realized there were tears streaming down my face. I got off of the scale and sat on the bathroom floor beside my old enemy. I picked the scale up and sat there with it in my arms. I cried and I cried. After having weighed over 300 pounds, and very painfully close to 400 pounds for almost a decade, my weight now started with a 1. It was an amazing moment. So many memories, most of them painful, ran through my mind. Hurtful things that had been said, names I had been called, memories of how I had been treated, all flooded my being with raw emotion. It's almost difficult to put into words the exact feelings that raced through my head on that morning.

It also dawned on me that when I lost five more pounds, I would have lost 200 pounds total. That was huge to me. All those nights that I lay in bed thinking it was impossible, all those times I thought it was just too insurmountable a number and a task I could never accomplish, all the years I had thought my obesity was an opponent I couldn't conquer, and I had almost accomplished it in 11 months. My goal weight was 165 pounds, because that's what I had weighed in high school. I was 5'9 with shoes on, and that's what the doctor's chart had said I should weigh. So, I sat there realizing that I was only 31 pounds away from that weight. I again thought back to when I had said that if I only had 30 to 40 pounds to lose, I wouldn't even bother losing it. I laughed as I remembered making that statement, because at this point, nothing was going to stop me from charging on to lose the remainder of my weight.

I was startled back to reality by my beautiful son standing in the doorway. It was early in the morning, and he had just gotten out of bed. He was rubbing his eyes, with a horrified look on his face. He said, "Don't cry if you gained a little weight Mommy, I'll help you lose it now that we're home." I realized I was still sitting in the middle of the bathroom floor, butt naked, holding the scale and sobbing like a lunatic. I asked him to hand me a towel. I set the scale down, covered myself up, and stood up quickly.

I told him to come over by the scale and I stood on it again. He looked down and saw the 196 and I'll never forget the sheer happiness and look of pure excitement on his face when he looked up at me. He started jumping and screaming for me. It was a beautiful, happy moment of complete joy that the two of us shared. He ran down the hall and was doing the fist-pump and yelling, "Yes! Yes! Yes!" As I remember that moment, I have to say that I'm not sure that life gets much better than that. This little boy, who had loved me at my worst, was now celebrating me at my best. He was genuinely and unabashedly happy for me.

In that moment, I knew every single thing I'd been through had been worth it. All of the planning, the waiting, the pain, the vomiting, the crying, the sugar deprivation, the hours and hours of tears and frustrations, every single bit of it was worth it to share this moment with my son. The years of lying in bed dreaming of being something and someone else had finally materialized into who I was in this moment. All of those daydreams had come true. God had placed a dream in my heart, and then He opened all of the doors to make it come true.

"The future belongs to those who believe in the beauty of their dreams."

—Eleanor Roosevelt

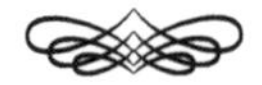

CHAPTER 10

"There is nothing more rare, nor more beautiful, than a woman being unapologetically herself, comfortable in her perfect imperfection. To me, that is the true essence of beauty."

—Steve Maraboli

My weight loss began to slow down as I inched closer and closer to the one-year anniversary of my surgery. I wasn't losing nearly as much, and as you can probably imagine, I was annoyed and frustrated by that fact. When I would go to Dr. Maguire's office, depending on how long it had been since my last appointment, I was accustomed to getting on the scale and losing 15 or 20 pounds. Now I was only losing 8-10 pounds per visit, and that just wasn't what I had been used to. I asked Kim how much more my weight loss was going to slow down and what I could expect going forward. She told me that I might only lose 5 pounds a month at this point, but not to be discouraged because I wasn't even at a year since my procedure, and with my particular surgery patients generally continue to lose weight for the first 18-24 months.

Kim saw the look on my face and she immediately did what she does best. She began to explain to me that it would be fine and I had to be a little patient as I was nearing the home stretch. She reiterated to me that I had already lost 200 pounds and that was an amazing accomplishment in only eleven months. She told me that I still had over a year left in that critical window of time, and that even if I only lost five pounds a month, I was still going to reach my goal weight. It made perfect sense to me on an analytical level, but I was on a mission to see that magical 165 pop up on my scale. I continued to eat right, to avoid sugar as much as I could, and to exercise. I really was a woman on a mission.

It was so amazing to look in the mirror and realize that I was a completely different-looking person. Sometimes while shopping I would catch a glimpse of myself in a mirror, and I would have to stop and look because I didn't recognize myself in the reflection. I remember walking into a Fashion Bug store in my hometown and going to the plus-sized section. The sales lady came over to me and told me that I was in the wrong section, and that my size clothes were on the other side of the store. She probably thought I was a little wacko because I just stood there, looking at her quizzically. It had hit me hard that a total stranger just looked at me and determined that I didn't belong in the plus-sized section.

I had tried to be invisible for so many years. I really had just wanted to fade into nothing and not be noticed by anyone, especially not when I shopped for clothes. I had long felt that most of society didn't see any beauty in my bigger size and certainly didn't find me attractive. Even though I had lost an enormous amount of weight, I didn't lose the inner scars that remained from living in a body most people found repulsive. People convey their negativity a multitude of ways. They may not be bold enough to come right out and say it, but they send passive-aggressive messages in a glance, a look of disgust, a comment, a sound, an eyeroll, a laugh, or a gesture. However the message is sent, it is received, loud and clear. I received those types of messages for over ten years, and I wasn't quite certain how I felt about the one that was just delivered by this innocent, unassuming saleslady.

In this moment, I wasn't sure if I was happy that someone recognized me as an under-size-14-shopper or if I was dazed because I was offended at her implication that the plus-sized section was not the section in which one wanted to shop. I had shopped in that section of stores for 15 years. This was relatively new ground for me. This was unfamiliar territory. For the first 22 years of my life I had been an under-size-14-shopper, but for the next 15 years I had been a plus-sized shopper, and even a super-plus-sized shopper for the last ten of those years. I wore a size 32, and before my surgery, some of those clothes were too small. But on this day, what I had never been before was an under-size-14-shopper, turned super/plus-sized shopper, turned under-size-14-shopper again. I realized in that moment that I had spent at least a decade on each side of that fence. I didn't know where I really fit anymore. Obviously, I knew what clothes fit, but I didn't know emotionally where I fit. Honestly, I didn't feel like I fit anywhere.

What I was greatly aware of was that I definitely felt some internal happiness at the realization that the woman visually sized me as an under-size-14-shopper. Why did her assessment of my physical size matter so much to me? If I was thrilled with my new weight and size, why did her opinion make any difference to me at all? Why did I base my feelings on how I appeared to a total stranger? Even after losing 200 pounds, one thing I didn't lose was my old partner in crime, the Homecoming Queen of Crazy Town. She was like tape, she stuck around, existing in the shadows, waiting to jump into action and reclaim her throne. She's not a bad lady. In fact, she can be quite entertaining at times. But she is a lady who thrives on misperception and in unrealistic situations. She makes poor decisions based on her insecurities, and while she may also wear the title of Miss Congeniality, she suffers from inherently low self-esteem. She will flash that beautiful smile of hers, and all the while be silently crying on the inside.

So, there I was, in a Fashion Bug Store, having the first of what would be many conversations in my own mind about how I felt and who I was becoming. The only thing I knew for sure is that I wasn't who I used to be. For the entire fifteen years I was overweight, I thought that when I finally lost the pounds, I would feel the way I used to feel. That was a huge miscalculation on my part. First of all, it was fifteen years later. My entire life had changed. I now had a son and a career, and I wasn't that care-free college girl anymore. But even more importantly, spending over a decade weighing more than 300 pounds had changed me forever.

My mom had always told me that change keeps us alive; it allows our spirit to thrive and to grow. I don't think I had ever fully grasped the true wisdom in that statement. As we each navigate the path of our lives, we are meant to learn many, many different lessons. As with any experiences in life, some will hurt, some will bring joy, some will bring us to our knees, and others will make us unequivocally aware that love is the most powerful force on the planet. Some tasks we will master, others we will not. But I believe, without a doubt, that in every trial we are faced with, we either learn a lesson or we teach one. Many times, we may be oblivious to the lessons we teach, but trust and believe that someone, somewhere is learning.

The lesson I was learning as I was finally winning my lifetime battle with my weight was that I had based every single bit of my self-esteem and self-worth on how other people viewed me. I was overwhelmed with the enormity of how absolutely ridiculous that was and it left me feeling sad and confused. When did I actually begin to place my value in the hands and minds of other people, many of whom, I didn't respect and several of whom I didn't even know? Who was I to think that I could even accurately interpret what other people thought about me and even if I could, why did it matter? Why was my self-esteem predicated on someone else's thoughts of me?

I remember watching Dr. Phil one day and he said to a guest on his show, "Don't worry about hurting my feelings, because I guarantee you not one bit of my self-esteem is tied up in your acceptance." I desperately wanted to possess that level of confidence myself. My mom used to tell me to "fake it 'til you make it." I didn't want to have to fake it, though. I wanted to actually believe that I was enough. Even though I had a very long way to go, I was beginning to learn that being confident doesn't mean everyone will like you. Being confident means that you know you will be perfectly fine even if they don't. In this area, I had my work cut out for me.

I believe that every stage that we go through in life has three parts. There is a beginning, a middle, and an end to the beginning, the middle and the end. For example, when a relationship has ended we can usually look back and identify a key event that represented the beginning of the end of the relationship. My realization that there was something inherently wrong with basing my self-esteem on the perceptions of others was the beginning of the beginning of a huge transformation in my life.

I've heard many people comment that they will never change after losing weight and that they will always be the same person they are currently. In fact, I may have said that myself. It wouldn't be the first ridiculous thing I've ever said. But there is just no way this is possible. There is no way you can journey through losing a significant amount of weight and come out the other side the exact same person. Even if you were the same person, no one else around you is the same. Remember Newton's third law: For every action, there is an equal and opposite reaction."

The person who was always your biggest fan, is now jealous of how amazing you look. The person who seemed to never support you is proud of you and has become your biggest cheerleader. The relative who always seemed to understand how you felt now thinks your cocky. The partner who loved you just the way you were is now jealous and feels threatened by the new person you've become. One of your very best friends says you're not yourself anymore. Countless people tell you that you've changed. People who looked down on you now want to spend time with you. Any time we change ourselves, it changes everyone around us as well. Some of the changes are difficult and hurtful to accept, and some of them are welcome and exciting.

I would never want to imply that the changes this transformation brings about are all negative, because that is simply not true. There are tremendous positive changes, and they are spectacular. However, I was rather unprepared for the changes that happened in my circle. There were changes that I never saw coming. There is just no predicting how people will respond. I can say, though, that by far, the most significant changes that occurred in my life, took place inside me. While I was slowly beginning the process of transforming internally, the rest of the world just noticed the external differences. That isn't meant to be negative. Many of the people who surround us don't really know us all that well, so of course all they are really aware of is the very obvious outer change of our physical body.

While I certainly endured my dose of mean-spirited people who used my weight against me, I also knew many, many kind, loving people. In fact, I believe the world is full of friendly, loving people. I have to address the fact, though, that many of those kind, loving people don't realize how they perceive morbidly obese people. I am not suggesting that those people mistreat heavy people or utter one unkind word to them or about them. However, in my experience a large percentage of those kind people didn't even notice or see me. It was as if I were invisible. Let me provide an example.

The people who had the seats next to mine at UD arena for the men's college basketball season were some of the most wonderful, kind human beings I had met. I thought the world of them, really looked up to them, and appreciated how nicely they always treated me. It was a family of four, and they actually had two seats next to mine and two seats somewhere else, so they took turns between their seats. As a result, I had gotten to know them all on a very small level. I guess I knew them as well as you can get to know someone who sits next to you at a basketball game. They were fun, friendly, and loved the UD Flyers.

The season usually started in November and since my surgery was in August, I didn't go to the games for the first month or so. As the season progressed, however, I went to the remaining games. Throughout that time frame, I lost probably 140-150 pounds. Not a single person sitting next to me noticed or even commented. During the last game of the season, a lady who sat several seats away from me came down to me after the game and asked me how I was losing so much weight. She told me that she kept telling her husband that I was really losing weight and that he didn't really pay any attention and said he hadn't noticed. She explained that on the last game of the year, she finally thought to herself, "This woman is absolutely shrinking, and I am going down and saying something." She told me that I looked great and she wished me continued success.

The people next to me, however, never noticed, and if they did, they didn't comment about it. I do realize that some people find it awkward to mention a weight loss. They are afraid somehow the person who has lost weight will take their mentioning it as an insult of some sort. At the time, I assumed that was probably why the people next to me didn't say anything. Fast forward to the next season. I had finished my weight loss and went to the first game of the season feeling like a new woman.

I sat next to my friendly neighbors and we were laughing and enjoying the game together and having the best time. Still, no mention of the fact that I had lost 243 pounds. It's kind of a big thing to not notice or mention on any level.

As the game progressed the man sitting next to me said that it was so nice sitting next to me because I was so much fun. He then mentioned that the lady who sat in my seats last year was very nice, but quiet and never really talked or said much. He said how nice it was to sit next to someone who loved basketball. He then looked at Lori and asked her where her other friend was and why she didn't come to the game. Lori and I looked at each other and had the silent eye contact that only best friends have and started smiling. Lori looked at him, then looked at me, and said, "That's her." He looked at me and he was simply astonished. He just couldn't believe his eyes. It was a nice moment and one that made me feel very good. To witness the shock and amazement in his eyes as he realized that I was the same person, was something I won't ever forget. There are some things that people can't fake, and he didn't even attempt to camouflage his shock and surprise. The essence of the entire situation was profound.

Later, however, when I was replaying those events in my mind, I realized that it actually was not only a little sad and disappointing, but also incredibly enlightening. As I mentioned before, these were very nice people. I would feel very safe in saying that they have never said a mean word to anyone. My point is that as a morbidly obese person, I was invisible to them. I never thought that I was quiet sitting next to them. I thought that I talked to them quite regularly. I asked Lori, who went to every single game with me, if, in her opinion, I had been quiet or reserved while sitting next to them the prior season. She said not at all. She said that she was kind of surprised when he said that, but she didn't want to mention it at the time.

What slowly began to sink into my mind was that if these wonderful, beautiful people who had sat next to me for at least a few years didn't really notice me or remember speaking to me, I had to have just been someone that they saw through or didn't even really notice. If that could be the case with these people, who I knew were wonderful, it's really no surprise that people who were not-so-wonderful could be down-right mean. That says a lot about the world we live in. How can an entire group of people be judged entirely on their appearance? I suppose it's accurate to say that is a problem that has affected many groups in our society for as long as we can trace back civilization. But as we begin to know better, shouldn't we do better? Obviously, I don't have the answer to cure all of society's ills, but I do know it begins with compassion. As the Dalai Lama said, "Love and compassion are necessities, not luxuries. Without them, humanity cannot survive."

I am a firm believer that if we do our best and leave the rest up to God, everything will turn out better than we could have imagined. I have always been taught that we generally find what we look for in people. Of course, this doesn't always happen, but if we refuse to feed anything but kindness, love, and compassion, don't they have to grow? I could spend a lot of time looking back and being upset and bitter about the many times that I was treated poorly, and sometimes by the people who loved me. I find that an incredible waste of the beautiful gift of life that I was granted. God didn't have to let me survive. He didn't have to let me heal, but He did. God clearly wasn't finished with me yet, so don't I owe it to Him to do my part in trying to promote compassion for the millions of people who are hurting and being hurt by the same intolerance and ignorance that devastated me? One thing I can say without any hesitation is that obese people are worthy of being seen, heard, and loved, and are certainly worthy of compassion. Kindness takes on many forms. Make a commitment to yourself to be one of them.

As the many lessons I was learning about life were increasing, my weight was continuing to decrease. In the last few months I had really begun to notice just how much skin was hanging off my body. I have to say that the body I was seeing in the mirror was not the body I had envisioned during all of my daydreams of losing weight. The more I looked into the mirror, the more I hated what I saw. I remembered that during my surgical orientation session someone had asked a question about loose skin following surgery and whether or not it had to be removed. Dr. Maguire's response was that usually most people who lost 100 pounds or less didn't need to have the skin removed, but a loss of more than that typically resulted in an extra skin issue that may need to be resolved. I had lost 243 pounds. Needless to say, my skin issues were significant.

I had skin hanging everywhere, and it all had my attention, but the place I noticed the most was around my lower stomach. As I was losing weight I kept hoping that the area that seemed saggy would get smaller and smaller, but instead it got longer and longer. I had a flap of skin hanging down from my stomach, onto the tops of my thighs. While this was disturbing to me because I didn't like the way it was looking, it also became painful and physically problematic. The skin underneath my flap would become inflamed and for lack of a better word, almost slimy. It also had a strange smell and nothing I tried helped at all. I was constantly washing it, pulling up the flap of skin, and putting powder underneath it, but it didn't make a bit of difference. I tried putting a soft piece of material in there to stop the two layers of skin from rubbing each other, but that didn't really help either. At my next doctor's appointment, I showed the loose skin to Dr. Maguire and asked him what to do to help alleviate the problems. He told me that the skin needed to be removed. I wasn't completely finished losing weight yet, and he told me the more that I lost, the more the skin would hang.

After Dr. Maguire completed my check up, Kim came in and we discussed the issue. Kim told me about a wonderful plastic surgeon in Cincinnati who did the removal of skin after bariatric surgery. She told me that she and Dr. Maguire had been quite impressed by him and his work. At the time, my mind was racing because I knew that if my health insurance wouldn't pay for bariatric surgery, there would be no way they would pay for the plastic surgery to remove the skin issues caused by that surgery. I hadn't even paid off all of the related bills of that surgery yet, how could I possibly afford plastic surgery? I tried to put the thought of plastic surgery out of my mind for the time being.

But my skin issues did not lessen. I think even more difficult than dealing with the large flap of skin hanging down over my legs, was the disappointment that I felt because I didn't end up looking the way I had hoped I would. I certainly didn't resemble the swimsuit model I had daydreamed of becoming for many years. Everywhere I looked in the mirror I saw skin hanging everywhere. My breasts had seen better days. They were really hanging low. In fact, they were almost to my waist. I felt like I had to roll them up and put them into my bra. In addition, the skin was very wrinkly and crinkled. I used to joke and tell my friends that my breasts looked like a pair of knee highs hanging down from my chest. They were like long, empty sleeves. My arms had a huge amount of skin hanging, and I learned from the people at the support group that those were referred to as bat wings. Oddly enough, the name was incredibly accurate.

During one of my early-morning water aerobics classes, I looked at my arms in the mirror and rolled my eyes and Alec said, "That's really gross." He was just an innocent little boy and he didn't mean to be hurtful on any level, but it still stung to hear that even a small child thought all of the skin on my body was unattractive. I thought to myself that if this sweet little boy who adores me thinks that looks bad, how will anyone else view me? While I was trying to work on building my self-confidence I was still a single woman, and of course the thought of being naked in front of any man was out of the question for me at this point.

Needless to say, I became an expert at dressing to cover up my skin. I had to tuck the flap of skin on my stomach into my pants when I got dressed. I never, and I mean never, wore anything short sleeved or sleeveless. When I would look in the mirror naked, I actually thought that I had simply traded one problem for another. Of course, this isn't true on any level, but that's what I thought at the time. I was healthy, I was enjoying my life, I was doing all of the things I hadn't been able to do in years. I always counted my blessings and when I would have those dark days, I would remind myself of these things. I'm human, though, and that didn't make me forget the fact that when I ran, my flap of skin would bounce up and down and smack my leg.

I mention the skin issue not to be negative, but to be completely honest. There are negative factors in every situation in life. In my situation, the negative effects of the hanging, loose skin were very minimal in comparison to the fact that I was healthy, active, and quite close to my goal weight. All of the medical problems I had before were completely gone. I was as healthy as I'd ever been and I finally had my life back. But what hadn't dawned on me yet was that I didn't really have my life back at all. I was actually creating a new one.

I hadn't really emotionally prepared myself for how the loose skin would look, what an issue it would be, or the physical complications involved. I wasn't devastated or depressed about the skin, but had I known what to expect, I would have probably not felt the way I did. It surprised me just how much I had stretched my skin, and it also surprised me that it didn't really look like skin, it looked like fat. I thought it would be paper thin, but it isn't. There is tissue attached to skin and so it's very misleading. I kept thinking I had more weight to lose, but it was actually all skin.

I kept the name of the surgeon that Kim and Dr. Maguire had recommended to me. I decided to call him and schedule a consult with him and see what he had to say. I figured that after meeting with him, at least I could develop a plan and move forward. I had no money and no credit, so I thought at the very least, I needed a plan. Even if I had no earthly idea how I would make the plan work, I had already proven that I was not a person who would allow that to stop me.

Determined to find a way to have this skin removed, I consulted a local surgeon, as the one that Kim and Dr. Maguire had recommended was almost two hours away. When I went to the appointment, I felt uncomfortable as soon as I walked in the door. The demeanor of the office staff was not welcoming on any level, and that made me a little concerned about what I was going to encounter with the surgeon.

When he came into the room, he had a young, very attractive female assistant with him. He asked what I wanted to have done, and I explained how much weight I had lost and that I wanted to have the extra skin removed. He immediately told me in a very short, curt tone that if I wanted to look like his assistant, I could forget it, that it would never happen. He went on to tell me he couldn't work miracles and I had to be realistic. The last thing he said was, "You will NEVER look like her." His words were nasty enough, but his tone was especially hateful. I was quite caught off guard by that comment and felt a little slapped in the face. I hadn't said I wanted to look like anybody. I simply said that I wanted to have the extra skin removed. His nasty monologue had stirred up a bevy of negative feelings that I had been working very hard to remove from my life. It was as if he were telling me, "You will never look this good; you will only be you and that is not quite up to par."

While I was fighting back the tears he started the physical examination. When he saw all of my skin hanging down, I could tell that he was somewhat overwhelmed. He started drawing diagrams on his tablet, scratching them out and starting over and then scratching those out as well. He looked like a mad scientist trying to figure out some complicated, mysterious equation. He seemed confused. I was definitely confused. In addition, I was quite concerned that he didn't appear to know how to handle my surgery. I did not feel confident at all in his abilities, and he had already gotten on my bad side with his dismissive attitude. He told me that I had so much skin that I would have to have two procedures to have it all removed. He asked his assistant to print me out an estimate, and I was sent on my way.

I couldn't get out of that office fast enough. I wouldn't have let that man put a band-aid on me, much less operate on me. This was my first experience with a plastic surgeon, and it was not a good one. I was a little annoyed with myself that I didn't confront him about being rude and condescending. The comment he made about his assistant was obnoxious and mean spirited. I really wished my confidence level was a bit higher, so that I could have said something that would have made him realize that he was out of line. But I was just beginning to possess the smallest amount of confidence, so I wasn't yet ready to stand up to a bully plastic surgeon with a bad attitude. I also worried if perhaps my loose skin was just so terrible that any surgeon would be at a loss as to how to proceed. I went home and dug through all of the papers I had from Dr. Maguire's office.

I pulled out the name of the surgeon Kim and Dr. Maguire

had recommended. His name was Jose Berger, and he had a thriving practice in Cincinnati, Ohio. I called and scheduled a consultation. When I arrived at Dr. Berger's practice, I was surprised how lovely all of his office staff were. Not only were they physically beautiful, but they were absolutely as kind as they could be. After my disastrous appointment with the other surgeon, I felt very insecure about this appointment. The last thing I wanted to do was stump another plastic surgeon with my huge flap of skin. It's rather awkward, to say the least, to stand, practically naked, while someone intently looks at the area of your body that you are the most insecure about. I didn't care if he was a surgeon, this process horrified me.

I was taken back to a nice room where Dr. Berger would eventually consult with me. This room had stacks and stacks of photo albums full of before and after pictures of his patients. The results were astounding. The sheer number of surgeries Dr. Berger had completed was unbelievable, but the drastic difference in these people's bodies and faces was almost miraculous. The previous surgeon I visited didn't have any albums full of pictures. In fact, he hadn't offered to show me any pictures of his work at all. Before I even met Dr. Berger, I knew I wanted him to do my surgery. Any surgeon can advertise and portray a wonderful image of themselves, but these photos did not lie. Dr. Berger obviously had a gift, and I wanted to be the recipient.

On a few of the times that I had attended the support group, I had heard horror stories about plastic surgery gone wrong. There were many stories of surgeons who weren't really plastic surgeons trying to remove extra skin with disastrous results. There were nightmare accounts of patients going to other countries to have surgery and returning home mutilated and in worse shape than they were before. A lady had shared with me pictures of her horrific overseas surgery and needless to say, she was beyond devastated. I felt so terrible for her. She was lucky to have even survived the surgery. As a result of their botched procedure, she was now going to have to have several surgeries to correct everything they had done wrong. I told myself that I wouldn't go that route. Even if Dr. Berger was way out of my price range, I would save up until I could afford him. I didn't want to have the terrible outcomes some other people had experienced by trying to save some money. The familiar adage of, "You get what you pay for," certainly applies to plastic surgery. While I waited, I said a silent prayer that Dr. Berger would be a nice human being.

When Dr. Berger came into the room and introduced himself, I was pleasantly surprised. Because of the Ivy League credentials he had earned and his renowned reputation, I didn't expect him to be so friendly and approachable. I was immediately comfortable in his presence. He was quiet and soft-spoken and had a gentleness that was compelling. After my last experience, I almost expected that Dr. Berger's office would be full of shallow people who were dripping with vanity. But thankfully, when it came to Dr. Berger and his staff, nothing could have been further from the truth.

Dr. Berger interviewed me, took a very complete medical history, and tried to get a clear understanding of what I was hoping to accomplish with plastic surgery. I told him of the complications I had with my bariatric surgery and how I had ended up on a ventilator. Dr. Berger immediately told me that he wasn't concerned about that at all. He explained that one very big difference between my bariatric surgery and any surgery he may do, was that he would be operating on a very healthy person. This made me feel good for two reasons. First, I was relieved he felt so confident that I wouldn't have similar complications, but mostly I was happy to hear him pronounce me healthy. That felt good.

Following the interview, Dr. Berger had me go into the examination room, where he and his nurse examined me. I explained to him that I wasn't completely finished losing weight yet, but that I wanted to get an idea of cost so that I could plan ahead for it. Dr. Berger explained to me that he didn't want to do the surgery until my weight loss was complete, so that I would get the best possible result. He then started to examine me and said that I needed both a horizontal and a vertical body lift because I had skin hanging all the way around me. I hadn't thought of that before but it made sense to me as he explained it. If I had that much skin hanging down in front of me then it was logical that there was extra skin behind me and on my sides, too. He also told me that I needed a thigh lift because I had a large amount of skin hanging there as well. He didn't seem overwhelmed or confused, he didn't draw a bunch of diagrams, he just stated what needed to be done, and he told me that based on what he saw, he thought I would get a really nice result.

I told him I wasn't interested in doing anything for my arms or my breasts because I didn't have the money and even though they were unsightly, they weren't causing me the physical problems that my stomach skin was. The assistant gave me the prices for the procedure and explained that I would need to spend the night in the hospital. Dr. Berger gave me a very reasonable price because he was going to do the body lift and the thigh lift at the same time. But even though his pricing was reasonable, it was still a lot more money than I had at the time. In addition, his price didn't include the price of the hospital and anesthesia fees.

I still needed to lose about 20 more pounds before I would be at my goal weight. I knew that would probably take a few more months because my weight loss had slowed down significantly. Dr. Berger's office had given me the list of some companies who financed plastic surgeries exclusively, and I thought I could at least apply for some credit with them and see what they said. Surprisingly, I was approved for enough to get the surgery completely financed. God again opened the doors I needed to get the skin that was causing me so much difficulty removed. I called Dr. Berger's office and scheduled my surgery. Like Dr. Maguire, because Dr. Berger was in high demand, he didn't have any open dates for a couple of months.

This was perfect, because it gave me time to continue to lose the rest of my weight.

A couple of weeks before my surgery, Dr. Berger's office staff called me and told me that a local news station wanted to do a special about the extra skin that is left following a major weight loss, and they wanted to know if I was willing to let them do the story on me. They wanted before pictures of me, wanted to film some of my surgery in the operating room, and wanted to follow me for the full six months of recovery after the surgery. I wasn't sure if I wanted to do that. My old insecurities were popping up everywhere, and I had a million negative thoughts racing through my mind. There was a great deal of silence on the phone while they waited on me to say yes or no. Finally, I thought about all of the other people in my exact same situation, or people who hadn't lost any weight yet, but were looking for a sign of hope. What if there was someone out there who thought, like I did, that they had too much to lose and that their situation was futile. That thought is what cemented my decision. If I could give hope to even one person who was walking that dark journey that I had walked, I would do it. "Yes," I said, "I will do it."

On the day of my surgery, I was very nervous. Even though I knew I was much healthier, I was still scared that I could have complications. The television crew was there, and they wanted to interview me before surgery. I don't even remember what they asked me, but I know I was scared. But I was also so excited that I couldn't wait to wake up. In the operating room, right before I went under, Dr. Berger touched my hand and told me "I'm going to take very good care of you Kelley."

The very next thing I knew, I woke up in absolute agony. I was in so much pain I couldn't believe it. I realized I was in my hospital room and I looked around and saw that I was alone. My mom had brought me for surgery, and because it was so far from our home, she had gotten a hotel room for herself that was very close by. I saw the button to push for assistance, and I told the nurse I was in major pain. She came down immediately, and I asked her what was happening. She told me that it was the next morning and that my mom had stayed and seen me in recovery last night and then went to her hotel. I had an IV that was attached to a button that I could push when I needed pain medicine. The nurse said that I hadn't pushed it all night, and that's why I woke up and was in so much pain.

Just then my mom walked in, and I started crying hysterically. I was in so much pain I thought I would be sick. The nurse told me that I needed to get up and go to the bathroom and move a little bit. My procedure was technically an outpatient surgery, and I wasn't permitted to be there more than 24 hours. I couldn't stay in the hospital much longer, but I literally couldn't move. The nurse and my mom kept trying to help me move, and I would just scream in pain. The pain was almost unbearable.

I moved the absolute minimum amount that I had to, and

still I was in agony. The nurse insisted I walk to the bathroom, and I screamed every single step of the way. Dr. Berger had left instructions with the nurse that he wanted to see me before I left town to go home, so I was supposed to go by his office so he could check on me. We drove to his office. Because he knew I was in so much pain, and it would be unbearable for me to even try to walk into his office building, he came out to the car to see me. He had his office staff bring out several additional pillows to put around me to cushion me better for the almost two-hour drive home. I had four drains hanging out of my sides and lower abdomen. I had on a full body compression garment that was incredibly tight and was supposed to control the swelling. Dr. Berger told me that he had removed eleven pounds of excess skin. I think this was the only time that I smiled. I immediately thought of what I was going to weigh now that he cut eleven pounds of skin off of me. After that, we made the torturous drive home. I clearly remember that when we pulled up into my driveway I just sat there sobbing from the pain. I had no idea how I was going to make it into the house.

Dr. Berger had suggested we get a recliner for me to sleep in. He had explained that my stomach muscles and skin would be so tight that it would be best for me to sleep in a more seated position. He also told me that I wouldn't be able to stand straight up for a few months because my skin and muscles would be so tight. He said this would lessen as time passed, and ultimately it would give me a nice result. Those next several days were absolutely terrible. I was in so much pain I simply couldn't believe it. I had drains hanging out of me everywhere, and my pain was off the charts. The pain from this surgery was significantly worse than the pain from my bariatric surgery. Every single day, my very first thought when I woke up was that I was in terrible pain. It just didn't seem to lessen very quickly at all. I will never forget that pain. Of all the surgeries I've had to date, this one, was by far the most difficult and the most painful.

When I would bathe and I took off the full body compression garment, I would swell so fast it was unbelievable. Not only did that add to my pain, but it made it incredibly difficult to get the garment back on. It was impossible to tell how I was going to look when I was all healed because I was so swollen. Dr. Berger told me that I had to wear the garment for six weeks after surgery to control the swelling. Initially, I hated that garment. As the weeks passed, though, it became like my security blanket. It was tight and I felt strangely secure with it on. I was becoming a little disappointed with my results because after about three or four weeks I still looked so swollen and strangely misshaped. I looked like SpongeBob, and was very square. My waist looked the same size as my hips. Dr. Berger explained to me that this was due to the swelling and that it would improve.

Well Miss "I want it yesterday" wasn't very happy with that response. It was a month later and I was still in pain. If I didn't stand up very slowly, I had outrageous pain ripping through my stomach. I couldn't stand up straight, or it felt as though someone was cutting me straight up my belly. I really had to be careful because it hurt in the worst way. So, to have all that pain and still look like one giant square when I looked in the mirror, didn't leave me very happy.

About five and a half weeks after my surgery, I was getting ready to take a shower one day, and I removed my garment. Just then, I caught a glance of myself in the full-length mirror and couldn't believe what I saw in the reflection looking back at me. I had curves. I had a definite waist and hips, and while I may not have looked like all of my daydreams, I was the best me I could ever remember. I didn't care that I didn't look like some swimsuit model, I was happy with what I saw. I no longer resembled SpongeBob, and I didn't look like a giant square. I was amazed at the body that was emerging as all of the swelling dissipated. It was sublime to realize that this body is what was trapped underneath all that loose, hanging skin.

The day that Dr. Berger operated on me, I wore a pant size 14/16. Six weeks after my body lift, I wore a pant size 8. That's how much extra skin I had around my body. The television station did a final follow-up show on my progress. I received a makeover, and they interviewed me one last time. Because I didn't live in the area, I had never seen the special at all. Dr. Berger's office obtained a copy of the tape and shipped it to me. Within five minutes of receiving that package, Alec and I sat down in front of the television, excited to see me on the news. They started out by talking about my story and showing my pictures at 391 pounds.

Then, suddenly, the unthinkable happened. There I was, basically naked, on television. I almost had a heart attack. I started screaming and carrying on like a mad woman. They had bars through my private parts, but still, there I was, mostly naked on television. It showed me naked before my skin was removed and naked after my skin was removed. As I continued with my screams, I looked over at Alec and his eyes were huge and his mouth was wide open. Then he just erupted into laughter. He ran into his room, laughing like a little maniac, and called my mom. I heard him say, "Grandma, we got the tape from the news station that did the show on the surgery, and Mommy is butt-naked on television!!!!" There were a few seconds of silence and then he replied, "Oh yeah, she's throwing a giant fit."

Two minutes hadn't passed, and my mom came charging in the back door. She just had to see this. Of course, she didn't think it was nearly as embarrassing as I did. She and Alec had a really good laugh about it, though. I guess it made sense that they had to show my before and after pictures to show the difference from the plastic surgery, but I just never really thought about all that would entail. I hadn't given it any consideration until this moment. I was never so happy in all of my life that I didn't live where those shows aired.

That surgery really made a miraculous difference in my life. Because of Dr. Berger's skill, I looked and felt like a normal woman again. I eventually did return to Dr. Berger to have the skin on my arms removed and to have my breasts augmented as well. I didn't feel like I was chasing perfection, but I just wanted to be comfortable in my own skin again. I actually ended up having several surgeries to fix some complications that arose because of my natural tendency to scar poorly.

A few years later, Dr. Berger referred me to another surgeon to complete one of the revisions he had started because he had to attend to his own health issue. My last few surgeries were completed by Kurtis Martin in Cincinnati, Ohio, and he did an equally spectacular job. I kept attempting to have my scars revised because I just didn't scar well. Some people scar better than others, and I was not one of the lucky ones. Dr. Martin finally talked to me about trying to achieve perfection. At first, I didn't want to hear his thoughts about this, I thought there was nothing wrong with me wanting my scars to be invisible.

Eventually I realized that he was right. Every time I looked in the mirror I saw something I thought needed to be fixed. It wasn't just about my scars. I hated my scars, this is true, but it went deeper than that. I would pick myself apart in the mirror and want to try to fix things that had nothing to do with scars. More than once, Dr. Martin refused to do a surgery that I wanted done. He told me that he was in the business of doing surgery, and that he wanted to make money, but that he wasn't going to do surgery that wasn't necessary or that wouldn't get me the result I wanted. Of course, I left there upset and disappointed, but I had to respect the fact that he was being honest and forthright with me.

On one occasion, Dr. Martin refused to do a procedure on me, and I found another plastic surgeon who told me that the issue would be an "easy fix," and promised wonderful results. Sadly, as Dr. Martin had predicted, the surgery was a disaster and only made the problem area much worse. Embarrassed and disappointed, I returned to Dr. Martin, who had to complete a second surgery to correct the botched procedure. There's a reason why Dr. Kurtis Martin is voted the best plastic surgeon in Cincinnati, Ohio, year after year. As wonderful as Dr. Berger had been in the beginning of my plastic surgery journey, Dr. Martin was even more amazing throughout the middle and end of that journey. I am deeply thankful for both of them.

Slowly I came to terms with the fact that I was never going to like what I saw in the mirror until I learned to love myself. In spite of all the weight I'd lost, in spite of the skin I'd had removed, I still didn't like what I saw in the mirror. When I first lost all of the weight I thought to myself that when I had the skin removed I would be happy. Then after I had my stomach and thighs done, I thought after I had my arms and my breasts done, I would be happy. After those surgeries, I thought when I had my scar revisions done, I would be happy. It was never enough for me. I was chasing something that was unobtainable. After all that time and all I'd been through, after losing 243 pounds, after having several plastic surgeries, after all of the changes I had made in my life, I still didn't think I was enough.

I was incredibly insecure about the scars that remained from the surgeries. Most people were left with tiny little scars that resembled fishing wire. My scars, in many places, were hypertrophic, quite thick, and noticeable. I was very self-conscious about them. I'm not sure exactly when it happened, but at some point, I decided I just didn't want to have any more surgeries. I thought if someone doesn't like my scars, then that is their problem, not mine. Would I even want someone in my life who judged me because of a scar? Is that the kind of person God would ever want me to associate with? Nonnie always quoted Elbert Hubbard, who said that when we get to Heaven, "God will not look you over for medals, degrees, or diplomas, but for scars." Slowly it began to sink into my head that those scars represented my survival. Those scars should remind me that God said my time on this earth wasn't over yet. God could have called me home, but He didn't. Those scars are indicative of the fact that I still had a purpose and something on this earth to accomplish. Isn't that in itself, beautiful?

"While they all fall in love with her smile, she waits for one who will fall in love with her scars."

—The Dreamer

CHAPTER 11

"You've got to be willing to lose everything to gain yourself."

—Iyanla Vanzant

As I continued the journey to make peace with my scars, I embarked upon a great deal of soul searching. While it would be wonderful to say I figured it out quickly, wrapped it up neatly, and then my life became everything I had ever dreamed, that's just not the way it happened. In fact, that's not even close to what occurred. In so many spectacular ways my life had improved, yet I remained incapable of silencing those old negative thinking patterns and the behaviors that accompanied them.

I read online that some people consider the date of their surgery as their new birthday, as that is when they feel that their life truly began. That's a beautiful sentiment, but I don't look at my life quite the same way. My life is a culmination of all I've experienced, both good and bad. While it might be tempting to push the restart button, it would eliminate many things that have shaped me along the way. The roadmap of my life has taken many twists and turns. Some of them have been terrifying and out of control, but they have all contributed to who I am today. Every place I've visited, every mistake I've made, every friend or loved one who has turned against me, each and every trauma I have survived, every wonderful hour I've spent laughing with people I love, has left its imprint on my soul.

I have lived through many unspeakable horrors in my lifetime, but what I have learned is that the presence of genuine love is the strongest healing force that exists. As I lost weight and became smaller, I would take down the older pictures of me. I didn't like those pictures, and I didn't want to be reminded of how big I used to be. I thought I looked disgusting in those pictures, and I wanted to replace all of them with newer ones that showed me with my new and improved body.

Alec, who is now 22 years old and in college, told me recently that it always bothered him when I did that. He understood that I didn't like those pictures because I didn't like the way I looked in them. He explained, though, that he always loved those pictures because they were good memories for him and he loved me, period. He said that it didn't matter how big I was or how I looked, that I was his mom, and he loved me. He went on to tell me that he didn't have bad memories of when I was heavy and that he never felt like he missed out on anything because of my size. He said that he was happy, and he felt loved, plain and simple. He demanded an end to the negative talk about those pictures because he loved the woman in them. The amazing, unconditional love he described to me reminded me of something Maya Angelou said, "Love recognizes no barriers. It jumps hurdles, leaps fences, penetrates walls to arrive at its destination full of hope."

Love lessens the sting of the difficulties life can sometimes throw our way. One day, long ago before my surgery, my mom and her friend, Carol, had come over to my house to visit. They were sitting outside on some folding lawn chairs, and I walked outside to join them. When I sat down on the chair, it broke under all of my weight. I crashed to the ground, with the chair underneath me in a crumpled mess. The plastic arm of the chair had broken and scratched my leg and I was bleeding pretty badly. Worse than the pain or the blood was how I felt. I was so embarrassed and mortified. I stayed there on the ground, on top of the chair, crying and bleeding everywhere.

My mom and Carol jumped up and tried to help me get off of the ground. They hugged me, said they loved me, and told me it was okay. Immediately they started blaming the chair, emphasizing how poorly constructed it was. They mentioned everything they could think of to take the spotlight off of my weight and the fact I had just crushed a folding lawn chair. They hurt for me. They were embarrassed for me. They would have done anything to make me feel better because they loved me. I've thought of that event many, many times since. It was difficult enough as it was, but if I had been with anyone else when it happened, it would have been exponentially worse. That is the difference that love makes. When we are in the presence of genuine love, difficult events are not as hurtful or intense, because we know our soul is safe and we don't feel judged. That's not to say that we don't hurt, but love provides the buffer we need to manage the pain.

Love can provide a cushion, but it doesn't heal the fractures of our soul. That responsibility lies on us. I had always been surrounded by love, but I had never done the work required to allow my fractured soul to heal. I thought that if I pushed forward, the pain would go away. There were hurtful events in my past that I thought I could sit on the shelf of my life and ignore. I actually thought I was doing the smart, courageous thing. I had a Master's degree in counseling, and I thought I was capable of living my life the way I wanted, in spite of incredibly abusive things I had experienced and survived as a child. I felt like it was as simple as proclaiming, "I am no longer a victim," and proceeding on with my life. I thought that made me strong and that I was reclaiming my personal power. In spite of all of my education and training, I didn't acknowledge that there is a big difference between ignoring your past and healing from your past.

With the exception of my physical body, I hadn't healed

anything. When I was 391 pounds, I felt very unattractive and didn't believe there was a man on earth who wanted to be my friend, date me, or be around me. I felt as though I fell short in comparison to every other woman, and I simply felt unworthy of being loved. I craved romantic love, and felt starved for affection. That is a very dangerous, very unhealthy combination. When we feel unacceptable and unattractive, we are very prone to make the worst decisions about very important things. We make ourselves vulnerable, and unfortunately there are many, many people out there who are more than willing to take advantage of someone's weakness.

The men I became involved with at that point in my life were perfect examples of this scenario. All of the betrayals that occurred during my relationship with Jeff had left their mark on my already damaged heart. I had already felt "less than" when I met him, so you can imagine how I felt after being told that because of my appearance and my size, he could never be faithful to me. I was insanely lonely, and I wanted someone to love me. So, when an option came along, no matter how inappropriate that option was, I took it. This terrible reasoning on my part ultimately added additional wounds to an already-obliterated psyche.

I had been friends for a few years with a wonderful man. He was handsome and intelligent, well-educated and successful, and a good Christian person. He seemed happily married for all intents and purposes, he was a very devoted father and spouse. Many women flirted with him and approached him, and he never responded to them in any fashion. He never showed the slightest bit of interest and always appeared to be completely in love with his wife. I used to look at him and wonder what it would be like to have a man like that love me. I thought that his wife had to be the happiest woman in the world. Deep inside I knew that there was no way a man like that would ever love me.

We were both trying to make some extra money and were working on a project together, doing most of the work at my little apartment. He had really loosened up around me, and for a while I had thought that I was losing my mind because it seemed as though he was flirting with me. I can still remember telling myself that I had really gone off the deep end now, and my intuition was totally off track because there was no way a man like him would flirt with a woman like me. One night while he was over and we were brainstorming what to do next, he just leaned over and kissed me. I almost passed out.

My mind was racing with so many thoughts that I didn't know which one to tackle first. The one that seemed to take precedence though, was that I couldn't believe this incredibly gorgeous man was kissing me. Every woman who saw him was attracted to him and here he was, kissing me. It didn't take long for my conscience to kick in and remember that he was married. I never wanted to be that woman. Jeff had cheated on me so many times during our relationship, and I never wanted to be half of any equation that hurt someone in that way. But a starved child is going to eat, even if it means taking food off of someone else's plate.

So that began a very unhealthy relationship that made me feel even worse than I did before. I didn't think that was possible, but it was. I beat myself up over that relationship on an hourly basis. I hated that I was involved in it, I hated that I was succumbing to it, but at that point in my life, I had nothing and no one else, so I clung to it. No matter how inadequate and unattractive you feel, if you are reading this book and considering becoming involved with someone who is married, or already in a relationship of *any* kind with someone else, please take it from me and don't do it.

The really sad thing is I actually thought I mattered to this man. I actually believed he cared about me. Of course he didn't care about me. He had always told me that he felt really guilty about our involvement as well, but he just felt so drawn to me that he couldn't stay away from me. I fell for that line of malarkey, too. When we are suffering so deeply, we believe anything anyone tells us that makes us feel better in that moment. Even if in the back of our minds somewhere we realize it probably isn't true, we hold onto it with all we have.

If you really think about it, dating this man was safe for my heart in a rather twisted, illogical way. I was living behind a wall of fat that shielded me from most people, and I lived in constant fear of rejection. How could he reject me if I knew

I could never really have him? If I knew he was ultimately unavailable, then wasn't my heart relatively safe? That's the kind of thinking that the Homecoming Queen of Crazy Town loves, in fact, it's right up her alley.

When the inappropriate relationship between us finally ended, it stopped because his wife had found out about several other women that he was involved with at the same time he was involved with me. He had told me that I was the only one. Needless to say, I was not, and as the truth would have it, I was about tenth down on the list. There were many, many others. I felt like a fool. I felt so embarrassed that I had been stupid enough to believe that this attractive man could actually look past my weight, find me attractive, and care about me. All of my worst fears were being reinforced by this disastrous situation: I wasn't enough. I wasn't pretty enough, I wasn't thin enough, I wasn't good enough for him to have actually cared about me.

I didn't have any contact with him for several years. Then, two days before my bariatric surgery, he called me out of the blue and told me he was divorced. I told him that I was having the surgery on Monday, and he said that he would pray for me. I didn't hear from him again until after I had lost all my weight. He called and asked to see me and I agreed to have dinner with him. His wife had divorced him a few years prior, and he was still single. The last time I'd seen him I weighed 391 pounds and I somehow felt that this was my chance to even the score between us. I had been deeply hurt by all of his lies. Even though I felt that I had deserved to be hurt because I knew better than to have gotten involved with a married man, I still felt very betrayed and used.

I sat through dinner wondering what I had found so irresistible about this man to begin with. He told me that he felt odd telling me that I looked beautiful now, because he had always thought I was beautiful, even when I was bigger. In spite of all the inner self-worth issues I was still struggling with, I didn't find him genuine or believable. As I left the restaurant that night, I wondered how I had ever believed anything he ever told me. I now realize that I fell for it because I needed to. I desperately needed to believe that I was worthy, and I attempted to fill that void in the unhealthiest way possible.

During one of my follow-up doctor appointments, Dr. Maguire had warned me about dating after my surgery. He explained to me that some women, after losing significant amounts of weight, latch onto the first man who shows interest in them because the attention feels so good. He cautioned me to not make this mistake and to first allow myself time to adjust to a new body and to a new way of life. He said that he had seen some very smart women make some horrific choices when it came to relationships, and it produced some pretty terrible outcomes in their lives. I immediately thought back to my own mistakes. I didn't want anything like that to ever happen to me again, and so I focused very intently on the advice Dr. Maguire gave me. He told me to wait on someone who was my equal and someone who was worthy of me to come along before I entered into a serious relationship. He called this his Father Maguire speech.

Another common mistake caused by inadequacy is trying to reconnect with people and relationships that didn't work out for us the first time. Many times, we try to re-engage with the very person who ended a relationship with us in the first place. I think this especially happens after we undergo a profound physical transformation. We tend to think that a partner who walked away from us before will want us back when we look better, but this is a pitfall derived from the old feelings that we're not enough. We continue to feel that our weight was the true reason the individual left the relationship. In my experience, I tended to blame every problem in my life on my weight. For every relationship that ended, regardless of why, I blamed my size. I never considered for a second that maybe, just maybe, we weren't a good match in the first place.

The important thing to realize is that if you tried your best and failed, it is probably best to just leave a broken relationship alone. Just like milk or meat, some relationships have an expiration date. When something in our refrigerator has spoiled, we throw it away. We don't dig into the trash can the next day and pull it out to see if it has magically become fresh again. We don't place it back in the refrigerator and think that by tomorrow, maybe it will be good again. But when we don't value ourselves, we have a tendency to do that with relationships that weren't good for us in the first place.

There is absolutely nothing wrong and everything right with realizing that you deserve better than what you've settled for in the past. As soon as you can begin to realize your true worth, you will expect better, and almost magically, better things and better people will begin to show up in your life. Unfortunately, this is not something you can fake. As difficult as it is, this is something you have to figure out on your own. Each of us has walked a different path, and as a result of our individual steps, we have different obstacles to overcome. No two people's obstacles are the same, and figuring out how to heal our inner hurts is something that will not be accomplished quickly or easily.

I continued to walk along my own path of self-destruction for many years after losing all of my weight. In college, I read the book, "It's Not What You're Eating, It's What's Eating You." I realize that at some point, as Dr. Maguire stated, after we've gained so much weight, our bodies can turn against us and make losing weight much more difficult. But the idea that this book put forth, and what I've learned the hard way, is that if we don't figure out and address what needs to be healed inside of us, we will continue to make horrendous decisions that affect our lives in very painful ways. In spite of losing 243 pounds, I remained every bit as broken on the inside as I was when I weighed 391 pounds. I was just residing in a different body. We can lose all of the weight that we want to, but if we have unresolved emotional issues that contributed to the initial weight gain in the first place, we are going to continue making bad choices while walking around in our newly-thin bodies.

I continued to date the wrong types of men. I dated men who lied to me, I dated men who wouldn't commit to me, I dated men who were womanizers, I dated men who could never give me the things I truly desired in a partner. Dating these men only exacerbated my internal belief that I wasn't enough. I was involved with one man who never told me I was beautiful, not ever. I finally mentioned it to him one day and he said that he never told me that because I already knew I was beautiful. He went on to say that everyone told me that I was beautiful, so he didn't have to say it. The interesting thing about this was that of all the people in the world, he was the only one I wanted to think I was beautiful. He was the only one I wanted to hear it from. Apparently, I was pretty good at hiding my true opinions of myself, because I certainly didn't think, and definitely didn't know, I was beautiful. Today, though, I also realize that was a form of manipulation on his part as well. He was withholding what he knew I so desperately needed, because it was his way of having power over me. If making terrible choices were an Olympic event, I'd have been a gold medalist. I had spent a lifetime perfecting self-defeating behaviors, and losing 243 pounds didn't change that in any way. I remained quite adept at doing things that would ultimately hurt me in the end.

When I wasn't dating the wrong men, I was shopping more than anyone should ever shop. I couldn't overeat anymore, but I could shop. It felt good to be able to buy what I wanted. For those few hours when I was in the store, I felt happy and good about myself. I always thought that if I could find the perfect outfit or the perfect shoes or purse, there was a chance everyone else would find me more acceptable and attractive. I would buy more than I needed and then not even wear half of it. I would charge my credit cards until they were maxed, and then stress out over how I was going to pay them off. I would shop for gifts for other people, and I would give to people who didn't even deserve gifts from me. I would give and give and give. I suppose I thought that if I gave enough, those people would love me. I never for one second thought that just giving myself would be plenty. I never thought my friendship or my love alone would be enough.

When you give to others without restraints, you set yourself up to be taken advantage of in the worst way. People who are takers and users become prevalent in your life. After a while some of my friends didn't even appreciate what I gave them anymore. They started to expect it. If they wanted to borrow money, I'd better come through with it. If they wanted me to pay for a trip, I'd better do it. They knew exactly what to say to get everything they ever wanted out of me. It took a long time for me to realize this, and it was one of my most painful lessons, but those people were never my friends. When those people showed their true colors, I was devastated. Eventually, though, I learned that not everyone you lose is a loss.

I was constantly searching for something to make me feel worthy. I wasn't a sad or depressed person. I was incredibly insecure, and deep inside I still felt as though I was never good enough. I managed to enjoy my life and to have many beautiful times with friends and family, yet I was never satisfied with anything I had. I always searched for more because I would hear that internal voice telling me that I wasn't enough. I wasn't as good as the next person. I wasn't as successful as my friends. I wasn't married yet. I wasn't any of the things that I felt I should be. I was a good mom, and I knew that, but I wanted my son to be proud of me. I didn't want him to be deprived of anything because he was being raised by a single mom.

I had worked hard throughout college. I earned a bachelor's degree in Sociology and a Master's degree in Counseling. I had always strived to do well in both high school and college. I was involved in a lot of activities, and I always wanted to excel in them all. This is so typical of someone who struggles with low self-esteem. They try to prove, through various accolades, that they are worthy. If you looked at the list of things I did in high school, you would assume that I was a confident, successful young lady. Nothing could have been further from the truth.

After my weight loss, I decided to open my own business with financial backing from my parents. The business started very small and didn't make enough money to even pay my salary for the first year. My mom worked with me and she also didn't take a salary for the first couple of years. I poured everything I had into that business. I worked nonstop. My son would come to my office after school and when I did go home, I was usually on work-related phone calls all evening. I worked so hard to build that business into something successful. Eventually that's exactly what happened. The business began to grow and to thrive. While it was still a relatively small business, it became successful, and we were doing well.

About seven years in, my mother passed away. This was a huge loss for me. It sent me into a tailspin of grief that I didn't handle well. I had served as a grief counselor at a hospice at one point, and yet I had no idea how to work through the massive grief of losing my mom. I had lost Nonnie in my late twenties and that was incredibly difficult, but I had my mom to lean on and help me get through it. When I lost my mom, I didn't know exactly where to lean. It was, by far, the most difficult loss I had ever endured. I had lost the one person who loved me in spite of how much I struggled in loving myself. My mom could always make me feel better and would always remind me that I was worthy of far more than I thought I was. She could always make me feel better, even if only for a short while. Losing her was something I didn't know how to survive. She taught me so many things, but the one thing I never learned was how to live without her.

My entire life I struggled with knowing where I fit, and after my mother's death, I felt more alone than ever. I was hurting and I was trying to do anything to escape the pain that my life had become. I couldn't figure out what the point of life was anymore. I began doing everything I could do to run from the anguish inside of me. Due to my surgery, I still couldn't use food as a comfort. I guess that was a lasting benefit of the surgery, but still, I blindly ran in the direction of any other kind of comfort I could find. I was so desperate to feel important and loved again that I began making all the wrong decisions. I wasn't intentionally trying to do anything wrong or nefarious, but I made terrible financial decisions, spent money in ways I shouldn't have, and didn't take care of the business I had worked so hard to build. So, it all came crashing down around me. My board of directors accepted my resignation and it was all over, just like that.

As hard as I had worked to have my bariatric surgery, lose the weight, get the plastic surgeries to remove the skin, and build a successful and thriving business, I worked equally as hard destroying myself. I was chasing something that had forever eluded me, and that was peace. The happiness and acceptance I so desperately needed would forever remain out of my reach as long as I was searching for it in places and with people where it didn't exist.

I lost everything. I lost all of my friends and colleagues, my home, and my career. Almost all of the people I had loved and had tried to be good to for so long turned on me. It's amazing how quickly your life can change in an instant and without warning. The people I had been overly-generous with abandoned me quickly. All because I was a financial idiot. In all honesty, I'd never had the financial expertise it took to successfully run a business. God had given me many blessings, but I didn't take care of them. So, I lost them.

My life as I knew it caved in around me. When the dust settled, I was alone amongst the ruins of what my life once was. I felt like no one knew my story. They didn't know how I had been hurting on the inside for many, many years. Internal wounds are so difficult to heal from, and nearly impossible for others to understand, because no one can see the scars. When you don't have a battle wound, people tend to assume you were never in a fight. I wasn't even cognizant of how deeply I was hurting on the inside. What I can say is that I made many mistakes because of the pain inside of me that was never allowed to heal. I was a champion at projecting my image as a strong, confident woman. No one had any idea of the secret pain I had been hiding for a lifetime.

Eventually, God allowed me to destroy myself. God allowed my behavior to bring me to my knees. All of the people who I thought really loved me had no forgiveness or compassion for me at all. They deserted me when I needed them the most and as a result, I was completely alone. But in my darkest hours, I wasn't really alone, because God was there. He never left me. There may have been times that I felt as though he did, but when everyone else ran, God stayed.

I questioned Him, I yelled at Him, I blamed Him, I tried to separate myself from Him, but in the end, I just couldn't do that. I would be so angry I would scream that I was never praying again. Two hours later, I'd be on my knees sobbing and praying. No matter what happened, I couldn't sever my tie to God.

After the dust had settled, God left me a couple of true warriors who stood by my side. I was perfectly blessed with who I actually needed. God gifted me with those crucial few people, who truly remained by my side and walked with me, even when it made their lives more difficult. Make no mistake, it was a very dark and scary time for me and my son. Sadly, he had not done a single thing wrong, but nonetheless, was dragged through this nightmare because of my poor behavior. But just like when he was a little boy, he held my hand and he loved me through it.

I began therapy to try to deal with the calamity that I had caused myself. I went out of state so that I could begin counseling with a specific therapist at her institute in Arizona. Before my flight, a friend told me to be honest during therapy. She urged me to share whatever had been attacking my soul for so long. She said, "Just be honest. Whatever it is, just be honest." I kept hearing those words throughout my flight, but I doubted it would happen.

I had no intention of being honest with anyone. I held tightly to the belief that there were some things that people just never needed to know. When I arrived in Arizona and started intensive therapy, all of that changed. I initially tried to resist, but eventually my soul erupted, releasing all of the pain, hurt, and devastation that it had been suffering through for years. I finally broke down and let out everything I had been trying so hard to hide from the world.

As a little girl I had been raped, brutalized, and repeatedly molested for my entire childhood. The abuse was rampant and severe. Relatives and family friends had stolen my innocence and destroyed what should have been a time of joy and happiness. My childhood was filled with monsters who were real, and escaping them was not an option. So, I did the only thing a little unprotected girl can do, I found a way to hang on. In the midst of all of the evil that was my existence, I found little bits of joy where I could. I was an excellent keeper of secrets, and that was not a good thing. When once, as a little girl, I attempted to tell someone what was happening, I failed to articulate the proper thoughts. I didn't have the capability of describing what had been done to me. So, the one small plea I made for help was ignored, and as a result, I never told again and the nightmare continued for years.

Eventually life events caused the sexual and physical abuse

to stop. Whether this was due to deaths or relocations, I was just thankful the physical torture was over. The fear of that abuse, however, was not over. It never went away. I lived day-to-day in fear of what nightmare I might encounter next. The insane thing is that I had an extremely loving mother and grandmother who were oblivious to the horrors of my childhood. I loved them dearly, and they adored me. They both are gone now, but they never knew the true extent of the atrocities that were committed against me.

Years later, when I was an adult, I could never bring myself to tell them, because I was afraid they would blame themselves, and I didn't want to hurt them. I guess, more specifically, I was trying to shield my mom from knowing that all of this occurred on her watch. I knew that if she knew the truth, she would never forgive herself. She was my very best friend and hurting her wasn't an option for me. That decision was a very unhealthy, inappropriate one, but unfortunately, it is the one I chose. As a result, my secret stayed bottled up inside of me for all those years. Throughout the course of my life, I had shared a few, minor details with a couple of the men I dated, but never the truth of the severity of my victimization. I couldn't do it. I was ashamed and terrified of what people would think of me if they discovered the whole truth.

I was a little girl. I was a victim. I was powerless. Yet I held onto the shame, humiliation, and embarrassment of it for most of my life. All those years I thought I was being strong by ignoring it and moving forward, pushing toward my future. I thought by achieving awards and doing well, I had overcome everything I'd been put through, and I was no longer a victim. I was a secret survivor, and I was stronger than what had been done to me. But I wasn't. That secret-keeping turned into crippling coping strategies that eventually became a ticking time bomb. When it finally exploded, it caused widespread devastation in my life.

My soul had been severely fractured as a child. During very important and formative years, I had been horrifically and repeatedly violated. As a result of that abuse, I had never learned appropriate ways to deal with much of anything. In spite of all the love that surrounded me, I felt dirty, unworthy, and broken. I certainly didn't develop any self-love or self-esteem. The strange thing is that as an adult, I would speak to people who had known me as a child and they would always say, "You were such a happy little girl, just a ray of sunshine." My little, hurting soul fought for happiness, even as a little girl. It craved joy and found it in the smallest of things. I don't believe that I was faking joy, I believe that in spite of the evil that monopolized my childhood, I found joy anyway.

But a fracture is still a fracture, and my severely-injured soul desperately needed to heal. I never gave my soul the attention or care it needed. As a result, I pushed my hurt down by eating, and quite frankly, food was a welcome and tasty distraction. I silenced my soul temporarily by finding comfort in food, and as a result, a lot of pain in the resulting obesity. When I finally had bariatric surgery, I couldn't use food anymore, and I ran from one destructive force to the next until I was finally consumed and ultimately frozen in destruction. My soul had finally demanded its due. It wasn't waiting anymore. It shut me down, and it shut me down hard.

So it is that in Sedona, Arizona, my healing began. I recall Dr. Phil saying that we can't change what we don't acknowledge. That was the first step of my healing, and that was the beginning of my new beginning. It has been the most difficult transition of my life, but at the same time, the best, and by far the most significant as well. I know I made mistakes and they cost me dearly, but those mistakes were made out of ignorance and pain, and were never intentional. God brought me to my knees. He allowed me to be completely obliterated emotionally and abandoned by the people I truly loved, so that I could finally begin to heal.

Because of that healing, I am no longer upset with the people who walked away from me. Had even one of them shown me the tiniest bit of compassion or grace, I wouldn't have hit rock bottom like I did, and I wouldn't have begun to experience the healing transformation that only God's grace can provide. As a healthier person, I am no longer upset with anyone, but that's not to say that I ever want any of them in my life again. I felt betrayed and stabbed in the heart. In taking responsibility for my own actions, though, I have to say that they couldn't have done that to me if I hadn't handed them the knife. I realize today, however, that I don't have to let people who betray me remain in my life. I can walk away and close the door forever.

Nonnie always told me that God doesn't bring people into deep water to drown them, but to cleanse them. My soul needed cleansing and healing, and I am happy to say that I may have lost everything, but throughout that process, I gained even more. I am finally emotionally free and getting healthier every day. I am learning to know, like, and love myself. I have learned that what I was running from was actually me. Instead of dealing with the parts of me that desperately needed healing, I ran as fast and as far as I could. Sadly, though, you can never outrun yourself.

God has a plan for me, and He has placed the people in my life He wants there for my future. I'm perfectly at peace with every single thing and person I lost, because I have complete faith and trust in God that those things and people were removed for a reason. God forgave me for my mistakes as soon as I asked, and I have been able to finally forgive myself. For the first time in my life, I have been able to claim the most important piece of real estate in the world, and that is the ground beneath my feet.

"Something very beautiful happens to people when their world has fallen apart: a humility, a nobility, a higher intelligence emerges at just the point when our knees hit the floor."

—Marianne Williamson

CHAPTER 12

"Never be bullied into silence. Never allow yourself to be made a victim. Accept no one's definition of your life; define yourself."

—Robert Frost

From the very beginning of this saga that began fifteen years ago, God has given me all of the things I needed and provided shelter in the middle of the terrible storms. My blessings have been many, and miracles have manifested themselves in so many different ways. My story is loaded with situations that, had they gone a different way, would have produced a substantially different outcome. During those times when I was at my lowest, God sent exactly what my hurting heart needed to be alive with hope again.

During my "collapse," I had returned home from what had been a very emotionally exhausting day, full of heartbreak and hurts, and I received a small package in my mailbox. There was no return address on the package, but what was inside was quite possibly the most beautiful and thoughtful gift I have ever received in my life. Inside the package there was a small box and card. This is part of what was printed on the card:

A Kintsugi Life...Finding the Treasure in Life's Scars

The Japanese art of Kintsugi (also called Kintsukuroi) repairs broken pottery with seams of gold-infused lacquer to make the repaired object even more beautiful and valuable than it was originally.

Most of my artwork is created with a Kintsugi-inspired process with polymer clay or stone pieces that have been broken and repaired to symbolize the way that the healing of the broken places in our lives leaves greater beauty in its wake.

When I opened the small box inside, there was a beautiful gold pendant with a dark red heart inside a gold circle. The heart had been broken into pieces and had been infused back together with a gold substance. It was a Kintsugi Pendant. There was nothing else in the box. There was no name signed anywhere and no other paperwork at all. I was overcome with emotion. Someone had known me well enough to know that I was broken into pieces over everything that had recently happened in my life, but also, that I struggled so desperately with the scars on my body.

This gift so perfectly illustrated the beauty that is inherent in healing. This miracle couldn't have been delivered to me at a better time. I was suffering so deeply and desperate for the smallest glimpse of compassion. Someone cared enough to find something so meaningful and have it delivered to me anonymously. To this day, I do not know who sent it. But what I do know is that it arrived, like all of God's blessings, in perfect time and was precisely what I needed.

Obviously, the wonderful person who sent this, knows me well enough to have been able to find such a perfect gift. If they know me that intimately, then I can only hope that they will, at some point, read this book as well. So, this is to that special person, whoever you may be. Thank you from the bottom of my heart. This gift was so crucial to my healing process that there are no words to adequately convey how much it has meant to me. May God bless you tenfold for your amazingly perfect gift of kindness and love.

Around the same time that I received this gift, I received an email from someone I didn't know. The email contained this essay from a website, United in Christ at Boston College. This was contained in the section of the website called Faith Corner.

Some years ago, on a hot summer day in south Florida, a little boy decided to go for a swim in the old swimming hole behind his house. In a hurry to dive into the cool water, he ran out the back door, leaving behind shoes, socks, and

shirt as he went. He flew into the water, not realizing that as he swam toward the middle of the lake, an alligator was swimming toward the shore. His father, working in the yard, saw the two as they got closer and closer together. In utter fear, he ran toward the water, yelling to his son as loudly as he could. Hearing his voice, the little boy became alarmed and made a U-turn to swim to his father. It was too late. Just as he reached his father, the alligator reached him. From the dock, the father grabbed his little boy by the arms just as the alligator snatched his legs. That began and incredible tug-of-war between the two. The alligator was much stronger than the father, but the father was much too passionate to let go. A farmer happened to drive by, heard his screams, raced from his truck, took aim and shot the alligator. Remarkably, after weeks and weeks in the hospital, the little boy survived. His legs were extremely scarred by the vicious attack of the alligator; and, on his arms, were deep scratches where his father's fingernails dug into his flesh in his effort to hang on to the son he loved. The newspaper reporter who interviewed the boy after the trauma, asked if he would show him his scars. The boy lifted his pant legs. And then, with obvious pride, he said to the reporter, "But look at my arms. I have great scars on my arms, too. I have them because my Dad wouldn't let go."

You and I can identify with that little boy. We have scars,

too. Not from an alligator, but the scars of a painful past. Some of those scars are unsightly and have caused us deep regret. But, some wounds are because God has refused to let go. In the midst of your struggle, He's been there holding on to you. The Scripture teaches that God loves you. You are a child of God. He wants to protect you and provide for you in every way. But, sometimes, we foolishly wade into dangerous situations, not knowing what lies ahead. The swimming hole of life is filled with peril, and we forget that the enemy is waiting to attack. That's when the tug-of-war begins...and if you have the scars of His love on your arms, be very, very grateful...He did not and will not ever let you go. Never judge another person's scars because you don't know how they got them.

I decided to share my story because it is an example of how we can heal our physical body, but ignore the rest of our being. Thankfully not everyone has experienced the type of trauma in their lives that I did, but anyone who has spent time on this planet as a morbidly obese person is going to have some type of healing to accomplish. It's an incredibly hurtful and painful path to walk. Perhaps your wounds are minimal, and if they are, you are greatly blessed. But for those of you whose hurts go deeper, please realize that they need attention just as much as your physical body.

If you find that when you lose weight, happiness still eludes you, figure out the origin of your pain. It may take some searching, but it's definitely worth the time and effort to discover the truth. Your soul has been suffering, and it's time for that to stop. There are infinite types of pain, but the good news is that there are just as many ways to learn to heal. Ultimately, you just need to start the healing journey.

Be a little easy on yourself. You've survived a lot, and sometimes we just need to give our hearts a rest. Remember, though, that you're in control now, and you don't need to settle for simply surviving. You deserve happiness, you deserve to be free from the things that were holding you back. You don't have to sit back and watch life pass you by anymore. By living for several years as a morbidly obese person, I missed enough of life. I don't want to miss any more, and I'm sure you don't either.

Throughout my healing journey, I finally began to feel that I was worthy, that I was enough, and that I deserved genuine love and kindness from everyone in my life and especially from the man with whom I was involved. I am living proof that you CAN heal and you CAN begin to love yourself. This letter was written while I was still in treatment in Sedona, Arizona, to the man I had been involved with for the last four years of my life. I have chosen to share this letter as encouragement for all of the people out there who may be struggling with a similar issue. Excuse any fragments or errors in grammar, as this is the original letter and I want to leave it in its original form without any editing. I call this, "A Letter From a Woman Who Found Her Worth."

You just don't get to be in my life anymore. You just don't. You truly don't want to be there anyway. It shouldn't be a big concern to you and I'm sure it won't be, but you will make one last valiant effort to show a minute amount of interest simply because your ego just cannot deal with me walking away from you.

Why do people walk away from someone? And why do people walk away from someone they genuinely care about? The answer is simple. Before I give the answer though I will say this. In the past four years, I could not walk away from you. Regardless of how terrible you treated me, how disrespectful you were, how downright mean you were, how selfish and stubborn you were, I simply could not bring myself to walk away from you. You were always the one who I just couldn't let go of and who I just could not get over. I begged God on countless occasions to open your heart to me.

God answered that prayer. He just said no. I sometimes sit and think about why in the world would I continue to even stick around a man who clearly had no true interest in me. Yeah... then it started to sink in. Me not being able to let go of you and not being able to ever walk away or forget you... That had nothing to do with you actually. Sorry to let you know, but it had everything to do with ME. As much as it will be shocking for you to know this, you were not so irresistible that I simply could not help myself. You did not have some magic spell on me and I simply became unable to live without you. That's not what happened.

No. As much as I'm sure you would love to think that was the case, it wasn't. There is a reason I continued to chase you and want you and obsess over you and make excuses for you. There is a reason why I always, always, came back to you and would beg you for another chance when you were the one who behaved poorly in the first place. That reason is ME. I couldn't get over ME. All of this chasing and obsessing and just feeling like I couldn't live without you was all about ME.

I didn't have enough love for me. I didn't value myself enough for me to say, "This is BS and I am walking…no, running…away from you. "I didn't think I was worthy. I thought you were so above me and that I should be lucky that you even gave me the time of day. But those days are over. Today is a new day.

Today I know that I deserve better and I deserve a man who will give me what I want and be just as invested in making me happy as I am in making him happy. I deserve to be with a man who adores me and treats me like that. We all deserve that. I deserve to be with someone who communicates with me because he wants to and there is no one in the world he would rather talk to before me. Because I am his best friend and he is mine.

You are not my best friend and I am not your best friend. You and I have done many, many things together and I have based the last four years of my life around you and I would bet my life you don't even know my middle name. I bet you don't know my favorite food. You have no idea what makes me smile or what makes me cry. How did my dad die? Any idea? No. Because not only do you not know but you have never cared enough to even ask a single question about my life or anything that has ever happened to me.

So at this point, on this day, at this moment in time in my life, I choose differently. I choose to walk away from this situation and to walk away from you. I have no ill feelings toward you and I have no desire to have some long, drawn out conversation, (via text, of course), with you. I don't need to be called a brat again, or be called selfish or spoiled or a baby simply because I have feelings and I know how to express those feelings. Our part in each other's stories is over.

We are two very different people and we both want two very different things from each other. And I have finally arrived at a point of saying that and being okay with saying it. You will move on and be with someone new and I wish you absolutely the best and all the happiness in the world. I, too, choose to move on and allow God to bring me someone new. Someone who actually can't wait to SPEAK with me, not text me. Someone who literally needs to hear my voice each day. Someone who wants to see me several times a week. Someone who plans his weekends around doing things with me. Someone who has time and space for me in his life and is proud to be seen with me and to say to the world, "she is mine."

You have told me countless times that you have your beliefs and I have mine. You've also said that you have told me since day one that you were not in a place to have a relationship with anyone right now, and that you don't even love yourself. That makes me sad for you. It truly does. But what I have learned is that you are right. If you can't love yourself, how can anyone else love you? You won't allow me to love you. You're not ready for me to meet your Mom. You, again, are correct. I should not meet your mom. I should not come to your house. You said your adult children who live with you would never accept me and that you don't want me to be embarrassed. **You** *are the one who should be embarrassed. The people in your world act the way they do, because you ALLOW it.*

So to answer the original question, "Why do people walk away from someone they care about?" I can't speak for everyone here, but I can speak for myself. I care about you deeply. You have made it perfectly clear that you cannot give me what I want. You have stated that you know the things you need to do to make a relationship work, but you are not willing to do them for me. I have heard you and I am walking away from you because I finally care about myself more than I can about anyone else, including you. As I should.

I may not know a lot of things, but I am slowly learning many things about myself. And the first thing I have learned is that I am okay. There is nothing wrong with me. And I love myself. So, guess what? You don't have to love me. You don't have to even like me. I got it covered.

Hallelujah. When I wrote that letter, I knew I would be okay. It felt wonderful and empowering to finally choose myself for once. On numerous occasions, I had felt as though I was stuck in the storm permanently. At times, I felt as though the dark clouds hovering over me would never dissipate. But as I heard Joel Osteen say, "Don't allow a temporary obstacle to block you from a permanent blessing."

I've reclaimed my life. As with every journey, the difficult part was to begin. I believe in my choice and in my direction, and I know that I'm on my way. I am greatly aware that when one door closes, another one opens and I choose to color my world with the warm light of love and the soft shades of *true* friendship.

Throughout my weight loss journey, I've learned that beauty doesn't begin in my mirror, it begins in my heart, and pretty comes in every single size. In chapter one I said that our bodies were simply a house for our souls while we were on earth, and my soul's house was run-down and condemned. After a long 15 years I now know that no matter how extreme the renovations to your soul's home have been, regardless of how beautiful the exterior has turned out, if the foundation is weak and unstable, you're living in a house of cards, and it is in great danger of collapsing.

Don't make the mistakes I made and have everything come tumbling down around you. While you're transforming the outside, work on the interior as well. As Henry David Thoreau said, "If you have built castles in the air, your work need not be lost; that is where they should be. Now put the foundations under them." *You* are your most valuable asset, so treat yourself that way and realize that if you're waiting for other people's validation, it's going to be a long, lonely journey.

I know how it feels to believe your situation is hopeless. But I'm here to tell you that it isn't. If I could make it, so can you. I gave up on myself so many times, but hope would never let me give up for good. It's okay if you fall. Rest if you have to, but get back up again. As tough as it may get, do not grasp onto sadness or anger, because if you do, peace and happiness will find somewhere else to reside. Don't you dare give up on yourself. I know you may be struggling and in pain, I was too. But, hope is only a belief away. I serve an awesome and powerful God. He opened every door I needed. Whatever your personal belief system is, have faith and believe in yourself.

This is my story. We might not all experience the same kind of pain, but pain is pain. We can't really compare one type of emotional pain to another. We have all suffered in our own ways. My pain isn't any more significant than someone else's. Whether your pain originates from deep trauma, or whether your pain comes from years of maltreatment as an overweight person, your pain is real. It is every bit as real as mine. We are all in the same church, just sitting in different pews.

Weight loss, and the resulting physical and emotional healing process, isn't a quick venture, but it is certainly worth it. Healing and growth is not the smooth progression many people assume. A jagged back and forth, similar to a bolt of lightning, is more accurate. You take two steps forward and one step backward. This can be disheartening sometimes, but if you realize this and expect that there will be some back and forth, you will be able to breathe, knowing the journey to wellness has begun. We all have doubts, and we all have fears that compound those doubts. The extraordinary thing is, regardless of what has happened in our past, we also all have the ability to begin again. No race is ever won without taking the first step. So, in those moments of dark uncertainty, just look into the mirror, stare straight into your own eyes and tell yourself, "I may not be there yet, but I'm on my way."

"For nothing is impossible with God."

LUKE 1:37

EPILOGUE

I recently read the book "God Will Carry You Through" by Max Lucado. One of the essays in that book, "In her own words: Cindy's story," says that if you look closely enough at the scars that Jesus has on his hands and feet, you'll see your name written there. Scars indicate the site of an injury, the place where pain was experienced, and blood flowed. Scars may also mean that you encountered something that could have brought you death, but you survived. In that case, the mark is a permanent reminder of the second chance at life you have been given. The essay goes on to say that we may have scars, but they should remind us of a life that we could have lost, but were given back. If we look closely enough at those scars, we will see that Jesus' name is written there.

I have slowly made peace with my body and my scars. I realize what they represent, and I no longer have any shame regarding them. I am proud of the way I have embraced my healing journey, and I look forward to continued life-long progress. Life isn't always easy and as one of my college professors always said, "We all suffer from the same affliction, chronic human imperfection." I don't expect or look for perfection in anyone else, and I have certainly stopped demanding it in myself. I have always been quick to forgive others and have finally realized it was time I forgave myself. I spent so much time trying to become someone else, when all I needed to learn to be was myself, my true self.

"Maybe the journey isn't so much about becoming anything.

Maybe it's about unbecoming everything that isn't really you, so you can be who you were meant to be in the first place."

—Summer Saldana

ACKNOWLEDGEMENTS

First and foremost, thank you to God, from whom all blessings flow. Thank you for blessing me with a life, saving that life (a few times), and giving me faith and hope; nothing compares to your promise.

Much love to the following:

A huge thank you to my son, Alec Gunter-Huffmon, aka, the Doodlebug, for always loving me; You are everything perfect that is in this world. I love you with all I have. You will always be my huckleberry. To Jeff Huffmon for loving me in spite of my madness and for being my family and one of the few people I will always love; To Lori Hughes for being the best friend anyone could ever ask for. I was lost without you and I thank God every day for bringing us back into each other's lives. I do not deserve you. To Chris Hughes for being an amazing husband to Lori and for tolerating and supporting our friendship; To Max and Gloria Adams for being a quiet reminder that the people who once knew you and loved you, still do. To Ron Hagen for being the best human being and one of my favorite people on this planet; You will always be my family and I love you dearly; To Brian Higgins for believing in me when I was at my worst and for loving me when I didn't deserve it. You are my family. 365/24/7, 10X10ND. To Amy Kelley for being my loyal friend and constant source of love and belief. I love you sister. To Holly Jordan for editing through all of my mess and not only making sense of all my emotional rants, but trying to understand them as well; To Sarah Butler for your edits and beautiful input and your soul which is lovely to the core. To Ginny Dowd for being a wonderful, loving person and an unexpected support; Thank you for guiding and teaching my most prized possession, my son. We both love you dearly. To Dr. John Maguire for being the best of the best and not only saving my life, but guiding me along the way of recovery; To Kim Hedgcorth for being the most beautiful, wonderful woman alive. Your patience and beautiful heart are overwhelming. You are a true gift from God. You will always be my angel. To Brooks Hall for being a wonderful Christian inspiration and a true friend. You will always be a member of our family. To Samantha Lewis for being a mighty, beautiful warrior who believed in me and stood by me; To Dr. Jose Berger for making all of my surgeries, your own work of art; To Dr. Kurtis Martin for all of your expertise and skill and for being infinitely patient with me; To Kathy Jones for all of your amazing skill for helping create my unique kind of pretty. To Tanya Schiering for being my brightest light in a time of darkness. Your friendship, love, and strength, saved my life on many days. I adore you and love you, and "Oh, FFS!" To my beautiful Doll, Carla Morman, for remaining my true and amazing friend over all these years. You are not only gorgeous, but you have an internal beauty that is inexplicable. I love you dearly; To Larry Moss, for being my source of strength; You gave me laughter and hope and stood by me when no one else cared; To Mark Zelezny for believing in this project and restoring my faith in humanity; if it wasn't for you, there would be no book; To Blake Gentry for your investment in this project; To Betty Volk for reminding me that there are beautiful people in this world and people who see straight through you and right into your heart. To Jeff Slyman for fighting for me and remaining patient with me when I know I was a real pain. You're the best. To Heather Cobb for allowing us to do our photo shoot at your home. And an especially deep, love-filled thank you to Leslee Vogal for helping me slay the monsters of my past and focus on the beauty of my future. You have guided me and continue to help me with my healing and self-love. You are a vision of loveliness and truth to me. You helped me find my life's true purpose and for that I will be forever grateful. To Lilly Putt, Jingle Belle, and Rocket Pop for being the true picture of loyalty and love; you are my very best friends.

God isn't finished with me.
The best is yet to come.

ABOUT THE AUTHOR

Kelley Gunter was born and raised in a small town in Southern Ohio. She graduated from a small rural school that combined grades kindergarten through 12 in the same building. She spent summers with her grandparents learning the art of true southern cooking from her grandmother, whom she affectionately called "Nonnie."

Kelley's love of reading was passed on to her from her grandmother and her mother, who were both avid readers. Kelley graduated from college with a bachelor's degree in sociology and a master's degree in counseling. Throughout high school, college, and graduate school, Kelley's teachers and professors encouraged her to write professionally. She had written both editorial and review columns for a few local newspapers, but only pursued writing as a hobby after the birth of her son in 1994.

Following a lengthy career in social services, Kelley began writing full time. Her first book, *You Have Such a Pretty Face*, is a memoir detailing the emotional journey of being obese and the surprising changes brought on by her 243-pound weight loss following bariatric surgery, as well as the emotional factors that contributed to her initial weight gain. Kelley is currently in the process of writing a second memoir, *The Homecoming Queen of Crazy Town*.

When she is not writing, she enjoys cooking, baking, and reading. She also loves spending time with her son, her best friend, and her three Rottweilers. She makes a habit of enjoying all of the sweet magic life has to offer and thanking God regularly for blessing her with the continued gift of life.

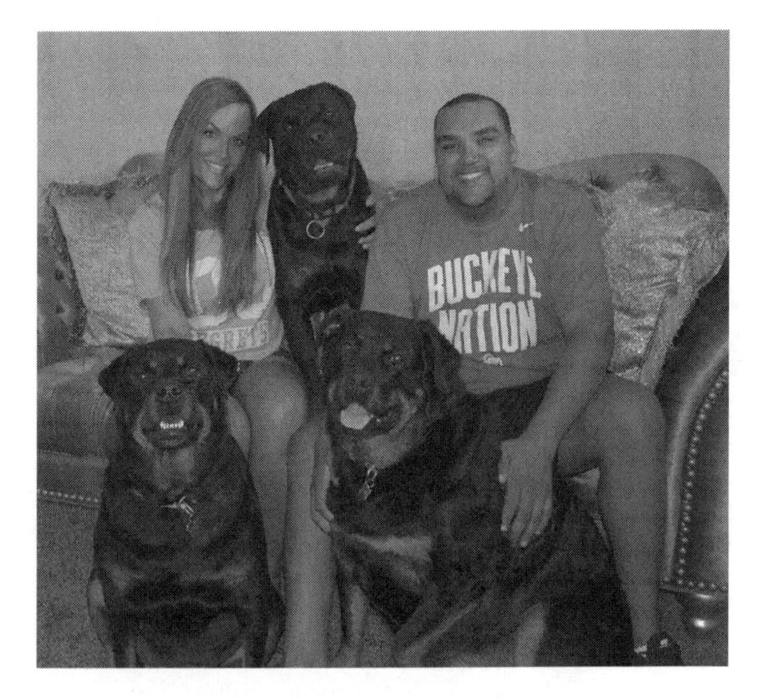

Kelley, her son Alec, and their three Rottweilers, Rocket Pop, Jingle Belle, and Lilly-Putt.

Coming Soon from Kelley Gunter…

The Homecoming Queen of Crazy Town

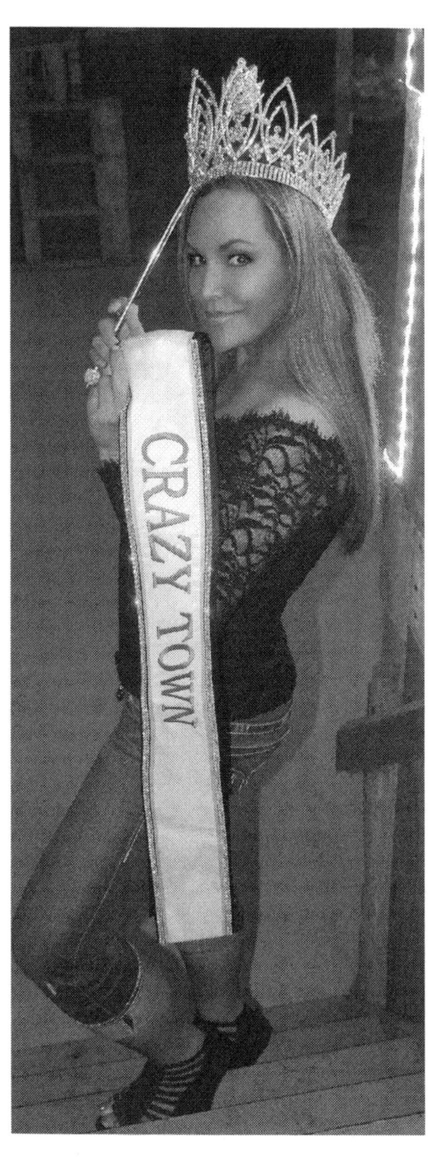

Made in the USA
Middletown, DE
14 May 2019